Natural
ARTHRITIS
TREATMENT

Maureen,
Thank you
for your
help.
Best wishes,

4/26/12

Natural ARTHRITIS TREATMENT

*The Buzz About CherryFlex®, AVOSOY®,
DONA®, and Other Natural Remedies
for Arthritis Pain Relief*

by CAROL EUSTICE *&*
SCOTT ZASHIN, M.D.

SARAH ALLISON
PUBLISHING COMPANY
Dallas, Texas

NaturalArthritisTreatment.com

Published by
Sarah Allison Publishing Company
Dallas, Texas 75231

Publisher's Cataloging-in-Publication Data

Eustice, Carol Ann.
Natural arthritis treatment : the buzz about Cherry Flex, AVOSOY, DONA, and other natural remedies for arthritis pain relief / by Carol Eustice and Scott Zashin.
    p. cm.
  ISBN: 978-0-9754060-2-1
  1. Osteoarthritis—Popular works. 2. Alternative medicine. 3. Arthritis—Alternative treatment .
4. Glucosamine—Therapeutic use.   I. Zashin, Scott J. II. Title.
RC933 .E846 2012
616.7—dc22

2012931813

First edition

Book project coordination by Nikki Stahl
Book design by Barbara Hodge

16 15 14 13 12 * 5 4 3 2 1

For more information about this book, go to NaturalArthritisTreatment.com

Dedication

From Carol Eustice:

This book is dedicated to my beloved husband, Rick, who was my partner in every way and a man who exemplified courage and what dreams can do. Your love will light my way; your memory will forever be with me.

From Scott J. Zashin M.D.:

This book is dedicated to M. Laurette Hesser and Terri Groom, whose advice and assistance over the past 20 years has been invaluable. Thank you Laurie and Terri!

I would also like to thank the wonderful librarians at Texas Health Presbyterian Hospital in Dallas for always being available to research my many questions about how to best care for patients. Thank you Cathy Nakashima, Molly Montgomery, and Jeanette Prasifka. Special thanks to Dr. John Cush, M.D. for his willingness to study CherryFlex in the treatment of osteoarthritis.

Finally, I am greatly appreciative of the hard work and dedication of my office staff in helping me every day in treating my patient's medical conditions. Thank you Courtney Brewer, Terry Crabtree, Chrissy Dickey, Kimberly Dotson, Evelyn Equizabal, Norma Kolski, and Maureen Rump.

Disclaimer

Natural Arthritis Treatment is directed to patients with arthritis and related disorders. The book is not intended to provide personal medical advice and should not be used as an alternative to appropriate medical care. The reader should always consult his/her personal physician before undergoing any medical therapy or changes in medical therapy.

Furthermore, if the reader encounters information in this book that differs from advice given by a physician, he/she should discuss it with the physician. The authors have made every effort to ensure that the information presented here is accurate as of the date of publication, notwithstanding that the authors do not warrant and are not responsible for the accuracy of information presented. In light of ongoing research and the constant flow of information, among other reasons, it is possible that new findings may invalidate data or facts presented in this book. In addition, dose schedules are being continually revised and new side effects recognized.

The authors, editor, reviewers, publisher and distributors of this book disclaim all liability arising directly or indirectly from any use or application of the information printed in this book; and make no representation, express or implied, that the drug/product doses, regimens, side effects and recommendations discussed in this book are correct. For these reasons, and others, the reader should and is strongly urged to consult his/her physician and the drug/product manufacturer's printed instructions before taking any medication or altering or discontinuing any existing medication regimen.

Dr. Scott J. Zashin has received research support from Cherry Capital Services, the manufacturer of CherryFlex which is a product discussed in this book. The authors do not endorse any company or product mentioned in this

About the Authors

CAROL EUSTICE has a Bachelor of Science degree in Biology from Cleveland State University in Cleveland, Ohio. Her original career path as a Registered Medical Technologist in a hospital laboratory ended after 16 years due to disability from rheumatoid arthritis. Since 1997, Carol has been a health writer, primarily writing for About.com (http://arthritis.about.com and http://osteoarthritis.about.com). She also authored *The Everything Health Guide to Arthritis* (Adams Media) in 2007.

SCOTT J. ZASHIN, MD, is a clinical professor of medicine, Division of Rheumatology, at the University of Texas Southwestern Medical School, Dallas, Texas. He is also an attending physician at the Texas Health-Presbyterian Hospital in Dallas. He is a fellow of the American College of Physicians and the American College of Rheumatology. He is double-boarded in internal medicine and rheumatology.

A native of Short Hills, New Jersey, Dr. Zashin earned his undergraduate and medical degrees from Dartmouth College and Dartmouth Medical School. He continued his medical training in Dallas at Parkland Memorial Hospital and the University of Texas Southwestern Medical School.

Dr. Zashin has published many articles about arthritis and is a sought-after speaker on numerous topics relating to both traditional and alternative arthritis treatments. He has been involved in clinical trials of both natural therapies and prescription medications.

He has enjoyed volunteering as the past president of the Lupus Foundation, North Texas Chapter, and as an executive board member of the Arthritis Foundation, North Texas Chapter. He is a frequent contributor to the Sjögren's Syndrome Foundation.

He is currently involved with media relations for the American College of Rheumatology and has served as a resource regarding arthritis-related issues for media outlets in the United States and abroad.

He most recently served as the moderator for the osteoarthritis press conference at the Annual American College of Rheumatology meeting in Chicago.

He formerly served as a rheumatoid arthritis expert for the Website About.com and is currently serving as a rheumatoid arthritis expert for WebMD.

He is very grateful to his peers for selecting him as one of the top rheumatologists in the United States by three organizations (US News and World Report, Woodard/White, and Castle Connolly).

Dr. Zashin lives in Dallas with his wife and two teenage daughters.

Contents

Introduction

Thirty-seven years ago, I was diagnosed with rheumatoid arthritis. My rheumatologist wanted to admit me to the hospital and begin some sort of intravenous therapy. What it consisted of, I couldn't tell you because, back then, I was uninformed and inexperienced. All I knew for sure was I had no time to be admitted to the hospital. Was that the best attitude? Not likely. Should I have asked more questions and considered what my rheumatologist had in mind? Very likely, yes. Would it have made a difference in the course of my rheumatoid arthritis? I'll never know. He started me on the next best, more convenient treatment with which I was agreeable. Could I tell you exactly what that was? Not exactly. I just can tell you that my treatment regimen consisted of several prescription medications. The day they were prescribed, I started down the traditional path of treating arthritis—with prescription medications.

Many years later, I'm a long way from being that young, fledgling arthritis patient. I was only 19 years old at the time—way too young to have arthritis. Or, so I mistakenly thought. Little did I know the day I was diagnosed that not only would I be an arthritis patient myself but also I would be the daughter of a man who suffered with scleroderma and Raynaud's disease and a woman who in her elder years would develop osteoarthritis and osteoporosis. I would become the wife of a man who also has rheumatoid arthritis. And I would have cousins who suffered with rheumatoid arthritis, osteoarthritis, breast cancer, and heart disease. The courage and strength with which they lived their lives could move a mountain.

Though several family members had arthritis or a related rheumatic disease, there were differences in the disease course and also in the treatments used to control the diseases. As for myself, I thought for a long time that my prescription medications must be the best approach.

I was diagnosed in 1974. Alternative treatments didn't really gain momentum until the 1990s. But by then, I had an attitude entrenched: if it ain't broke, don't fix it. I was settled into my prescription medication regimen and not about to be budged off track. I had no interest in learning about alternative treatments. Nevertheless, when alternative treatment became increasingly popular and headlines caught my attention almost daily, I was forced to take notice.

What could be so bad about alternative treatments, after all? If it's all natural, it must be safer, right? Or, if its use can correct a deficiency, how can that be bad? It was time to learn about supplements and natural treatments. And I did.

Before you can learn about individual supplements, you must know the difference between a drug and a dietary supplement. We need only look as far as the FDA (U.S. Food and Drug Administration) to understand the distinction. The FDA states that drugs are "intended for use in the diagnosis, cure, mitigation, treatment, or prevention of disease in man or other animals."[1] A dietary supplement is a product taken by mouth that contains a dietary ingredient intended to supplement the diet. The "dietary ingredients" may include vitamins, minerals, herbs, or other botanicals, amino acids, and substances such as enzymes, organ tissues, glandulars, and metabolites. The intent is to "supplement," not to be taken alone or as a substitution for food or drugs.[2]

Carol Eustice, author, writer for About.com
(http://arthritis.about.com and http://osteoarthritis.about.com)

---

1   FDA, "Classification of Products as Drugs and Devices and Additional Product Classification Issues" (June 20, 2011), http://www.fda.gov/RegulatoryInformation/Guidances/ucm258946.htm.

2   FDA, "Overview of Dietary Supplements" (October 14, 2009), http://www.fda.gov/Food/DietarySupplements/ConsumerInformation/ucm110417.htm.

CHAPTER 1

Osteoarthritis Basics

It's the most common type of arthritis. It's the type people think of when they hear the word "arthritis"—even though there really are 100 different types of arthritis. It is a painful joint disease that can severely limit daily activity and quality of life. It affects more than 27 million Americans. *It* is osteoarthritis.

Osteoarthritis is not a minor condition—it can have serious consequences. Osteoarthritis can lead to disability that can interfere with your ability to work and be productive. The end stage of osteoarthritis for many people is joint surgery, necessary to keep them functioning. But it's very important to understand treatment options that prevent that stage as long as possible.

According to the Centers for Disease Control and Prevention, there are significant social and economic costs related to osteoarthritis. In the next 20 years, the number of people affected by osteoarthritis, the impact on their health, and the economic consequences of the disease are expected to increase—dramatically. Because of the individual impact of osteoarthritis and its impact on society, understanding the disease and finding the most effective treatment are essential.

WHAT CAUSES OSTEOARTHRITIS?

Osteoarthritis is caused by the breakdown or wearing away of cartilage in one or more joints. Normal cartilage is a hard, smooth, slippery tissue that covers the ends of the bones that form a joint. Cartilage serves as a cushion or shock absorber and allows the bones to glide over one another painlessly.

When cartilage loss occurs, the bones of the joint become rough rather than smooth. The deterioration can become so severe that eventually there is no cushion and bone rubs against bone. There also can be changes in structures around the joint (such as muscles and tendons), fluid accumulation, and development of bone spurs (bony outgrowth). When that occurs, chronic pain and sometimes loss of mobility and disability follow.

WHAT CAUSES THE BREAKDOWN OF CARTILAGE?

Cartilage is composed of 65% to 80% water, collagen (fibrous proteins), proteoglycans (proteins and sugars that interweave with collagen), and chondrocytes (cells that produce cartilage). A decrease in cartilage volume and thickness occurs with cartilage loss, causing the joint space to narrow. Maximum joint space narrowing causes bone to rub on bone.

It has been hard to pinpoint exactly what causes cartilage loss. Experts do suggest it is due to both mechanical and molecular factors.[1] As an example, joint injury is a mechanical factor that contributes to cartilage loss, including meniscus tears. There are two menisci in your knee that rest between your thigh and your shin bone. These C-shaped pieces of cartilage act as shock absorbers to cushion the joint.

Synovitis (inflammation of the lining of your joint) and joint effusion (fluid) are also predictors of cartilage loss. Being overweight is also a risk factor. In one study, researchers concluded that with a one-unit increase in BMI (body mass index), the odds of rapid cartilage loss increase by 11%.[2]

SYMPTOMS

It is possible for you to have visible joint damage on x-ray but few, if any, symptoms to go along with it. The opposite is also true: it's possible to have pain or other osteoarthritis symptoms but no evidence of the disease on x-ray.

Common symptoms associated with osteoarthritis include:

- Joint pain
- Joint stiffness
- Joint tenderness
- Limited range of motion
- Crepitus (grinding sensation with movement)
- Joint effusion (fluid)
- Local inflammation (redness and warmth)
- Bony enlargements (bone spurs)

---

1   Centers for Disease Control and Prevention, "Osteoarthritis" (June 25, 2010), http://www. cdc.gov/arthritis/basics/osteoarthritis.htm.

2   Frank W. Roemer, MD, et al., "Risk Factors for MRI-Detected Rapid Cartilage Loss of the Tibio-femoral Joint over a 30-Month Period: The MOST Study," *Radiology* 252 (September 2009): 772–780. Published online July 27, 2009, doi:10.1148/radiol.2523082197.

As you see, pain tops the list of symptoms. Osteoarthritis pain usually develops gradually, and symptoms usually are localized to the affected joint. With mild to moderate osteoarthritis, pain worsens with use of the joint or overuse, and it improves with rest. As osteoarthritis pain becomes more severe, there is decreased physical function and increased disability, which means that activities of daily living, work, and leisure all become difficult.

DIAGNOSIS

When diagnosing osteoarthritis, your doctor must first distinguish the symptoms you are experiencing from those associated with other types of arthritis. Your **medical history** is of particular importance. Along with information about past medical conditions, allergies, treatments, and surgical procedures, your doctor will focus on your current medical status. Your doctor will want to know whether you injured the joint, whether your symptoms came about suddenly or gradually, what causes them to worsen, and whether the symptoms are limited to that joint. Patients with osteoarthritis often complain of joint discomfort or stiffness on awakening that lasts less than 30 minutes. This amount of morning stiffness differs from inflammatory types of arthritis such as lupus or rheumatoid arthritis that may last 1-2 hours.

The medical history will be followed by a **physical examination**. Your doctor will observe you for any of the visible signs and symptoms of osteoarthritis. Your doctor will also examine each joint for its range of motion.

X-rays or other imaging studies are typically ordered and used to find evidence to support the diagnosis of osteoarthritis. Images show the degree of joint space narrowing, as well as any evidence of bony outgrowth, also called spurs. Last but not least, **laboratory tests** are utilized primarily to rule out other types of arthritis.

KNOW YOUR TREATMENT OPTIONS

It's important for you to learn about the various treatment options for osteoarthritis. It will take trial and error to determine what works best for you. Initially, it's not uncommon for a patient to be prescribed a pain medication and/or an anti-inflammatory drug. It's actually appropriate, because you and your doctor are looking for quick results.

Perhaps medication will have a permanent place in your treatment regimen, but there are other treatments that deserve your consideration, especially for long-term management of osteoarthritis. There are nondrug treatment options and natural options that you should know about. As you try to avoid side effects associated with long-term use of medications or the need for last-resort joint surgery, a look at nondrug treatments would seem useful.

Nondrug Treatment Options

The latest version of nondrug treatment guidelines for hand, hip, and knee osteoarthritis was released in 2000 by the American College of Rheumatology. That's well over a decade ago. It was updated in 2005, following the withdrawal of the arthritis medication Vioxx from the market.

A technical panel of experts began revising those guidelines for the nondrug treatment of hand, hip, and knee osteoarthritis in 2008. The proposed revisions are currently under review by the American College of Rheumatology, and the expectation is that they will be published soon. The panel reportedly found strong evidence that exercise and weight control have a profound impact on managing hip and knee osteoarthritis. While we await the revisions, let's look at some of the current guidelines.

16 Components of Nondrug Treatment Guidelines for Hip and Knee Osteoarthritis

Patient education

Self-management programs (e.g., Arthritis Foundation Self-Management Program)

Personalized social support through telephone contact

Weight loss (if overweight)

Aerobic exercise programs

Physical therapy

Range-of-motion exercises

Muscle-strengthening exercises

Assistive devices for ambulation

Patellar taping

Appropriate footwear

Lateral-wedged insoles

Bracing

Occupational therapy

Joint protection and energy conservation

Assistive devices for activities of daily living

Remember that you may find some of these more effective than others. The nondrug treatments for osteoarthritis focus on teaching you about the disease, building strength, managing symptoms, protecting your joints, and living well despite your physical limitations. Each nondrug treatment recommendation is not to be viewed as a solution, sole and separate. They can be effective in combination. Let's consider what the experts said about each component.[3]

Patient education

We can't say it enough: it's imperative that you learn all that you can about osteoarthritis. You need to understand your disease to be able to follow what your doctor tells you, just as you need to know what is important to tell or ask your doctor. Some patients believe it's the doctor's job to direct their treatment plan. Certainly, your doctor's advice and recommendations are invaluable. But your doctor is not with you 24-7, and it is your responsibility to understand both good and bad aspects of your treatment. You should be able to discuss with your doctor the effectiveness or ineffectiveness of your current treatment as compared with what it is expected to do for you. If family, friends, or caregivers are involved in your treatment, they should also be educated about the disease and treatment, to the degree that is appropriate.

---

3   American College of Rheumatology, "Practice Guidelines: Recommendations for the Medical Management of Osteoarthritis of the Hip and Knee" (May 12, 2000), http://www.rheumatology.org/practice/clinical/guidelines/oa-mgmt.asp

Self-management programs (e.g., Arthritis Foundation Self-Management Program)

Participation in self-management programs, such as the Arthritis Foundation Self-Management Program, reportedly is associated with decreased joint pain, decreased frequency of arthritis-related doctor visits, increased physical activity, and over-all improvement in quality of life.[4] Self-management programs focus on giving you the techniques and skills you need to manage osteoarthritis. Elements of the program may include pain management, relaxation techniques, stress management, biofeedback, and regular exercise. Self-management programs can consist of one-on-one instruction, reading materials, or classes. It's all designed to guide you toward actions that help you help yourself.

Personalized social support through telephone contact

Communication is just as important as education, according to studies. Interestingly, it has been shown that personalized social support, either directly or by periodic telephone contact, is a cost-effective nondrug treatment for osteoarthritis. One study showed that monthly telephone calls by trained nonmedical personnel to discuss things such as joint pain, medications, drug side effects, compliance with treatment, and upcoming appointments were related to improvement in joint pain and joint function without a big increase in treatment cost.[5]

---

4   E. Superio-Cabuslay et al., "Patient Education Interventions in Osteoarthritis and Rheumatoid Arthritis: A Meta-Analytic Comparison with Nonsteroidal Anti-Inflammatory Drug Treatment," *Arthritis Care and Research 9* (1996): 292–301.

5   M. Weinberger et al., "Cost-Effectiveness of Increased Telephone Contact for Patients with Osteoarthritis: A Randomized, Controlled Trial." *Arthritis and Rheumatism 36* (1993): 243–246.

Weight loss (if overweight)

Much has been written and reported about the positive effect of maintaining your ideal weight as it relates to the management of osteoarthritis. It is known that being over-weight adds burden and stress to your weight-bearing joints, which in turn worsens joint function and hastens disability. In February 2010, the Centers for Disease Control and Prevention and the Arthritis Foundation announced *A National Public Health Agenda for Osteoarthritis*, a major initiative with goals to help people living with osteoarthritis. Weight management is a major component of the initiative.

People with knee osteoarthritis who achieve just modest weight loss can improve their physical function, self-reported level of disability, pain, and quality of life. Are you wondering how modest weight loss can do all of that? Overweight and obese adults with knee osteoarthritis who lose one pound reduce knee joint load fourfold. According to the initiative, zeroing in on programs that promote healthy eating and regular physical activity will help you achieve your weight goals.[6]

Aerobic exercise programs

According to the initiative, low-impact, moderate-intensity aerobic physical activity should be promoted for adults with osteoarthritis of the hip and knee. Aerobic means "with air or oxygen." Aerobic exercise is exercise performed at an intensity that allows the cardiovascular system to supply the

---

6   CDC and Arthritis Foundation, "A National Public Health Agenda for Osteoarthritis" (February 2010), http://www.cdc.gov/arthritis/docs/OAagenda.pdf.

muscles with sufficient oxygen. Specifically, it refers to low-impact exercise done continuously (such as walking, swimming, or cycling) in order to elevate your heart rate to 70% or 80% of your maximum heart rate. Aerobic exercise or activity helps build endurance and burn calories, too.

Physical therapy

Physical therapy plays a major role in helping osteoarthritis patients with functional limitations. A physical therapist can evaluate your joints for strength, stability, and mobility. The therapist then can create an appropriate exercise program for the purpose of improving range of motion and improving strength in the muscles that surround the joints.

Physical therapists also instruct patients about the use of assistive devices. Mobility devices (assistive devices for mobility) include canes, crutches, or walkers. Hold the cane in the hand opposite from the affected knee or hip. The therapists also focus on the benefits of joint protection, energy conservation, the use of splints, and other assistive devices. There are many!

Range-of-motion exercises

Range of motion refers to the distance and direction a joint can move to its full potential. Each joint has a normal range of motion. "Limited" range of motion refers to a joint that has less than normal movement. The limited motion can interfere with usual activities.

Range-of-motion exercises gently work the existing range of motion by moving the joint through its full range. As range of motion improves, pain, swelling, and stiffness decrease.

At first, your therapist or the use of some gym equipment can passively move you through the range of motion. No effort is required of you, which is why it is called passive range-of-motion exercise. The next step up would have you doing the range-of-motion exercises with some help from your therapist (active assistive range-of-motion exercise). Finally, you're on your own, performing range-of-motion exercises without assistance (active range-of-motion exercise).

Muscle-strengthening exercises

While aerobic exercise offers many health benefits, it does not make your muscles strong—strength training does. Strengthening exercises can help you maintain or increase muscle strength. Strong muscles help support and protect joints affected by osteoarthritis. It's actually that simple.

Tufts University completed a strength-training program with older men and women with moderate to severe knee osteoarthritis. It was a 16-week program, and results showed that strength training decreased pain by 43%, increased muscle strength and general physical performance, improved the signs and symptoms of osteoarthritis, and decreased disability. Easing osteoarthritis pain through strength training was viewed as just as effective, if not more effective, than medications.

Assistive devices for ambulation

Ambulation means walking, so this recommendation looks to any or all assistive devices that help you walk. Assistive devices for ambulation include canes, crutches, or walkers, which take stress off of your joints while improving balance and steadying your gait. When using a cane, hold it in the hand on the opposite side of the affected knee or hip. Electric scooters are an option when ambulation becomes difficult.

Patellar taping

The application and positioning of tape to align the knee in a more stable position is known as knee taping or patellar taping. The more stable alignment can reduce stress on the soft tissues that surround the knee and reduce osteoarthritis symptoms. Precise position of the tape is important to properly unload stress from specific knee components.

Appropriate footwear

Your choice of footwear can affect the load or stress put on your knee joint and consequently impact knee osteoarthritis. High-heel shoes increase the force across the patello-femoral component of the knee (behind the kneecap) and the compressive force on the medial compartment of the knee (the inside of the knee). Researchers in one study concluded that the additional force from wearing high-heel shoes may result in degenerative changes to the knee.

In another study, involving healthy young women and healthy elderly women, women's dress shoes with moderate heel height were evaluated. Results showed that even shoes with a moderate heel significantly increased force across the knee joint.

Finally, a study compared the use of walking shoes to going barefoot. Joint loads at the hips and knees significantly decreased during barefoot walking. Some recommended shoe brands include Rockport, Easy Spirit, and SAS.

Lateral-wedged insoles

A lateral-wedge insole can be worn inside of your shoe. A lateral-wedge insole is thinner at the instep and thicker at the outer edge of the foot. The angle of the lateral-wedge insole can be customized. Lateral-wedge insoles alter knee biomechanics during walking by reducing what is known as varus torque (twisting of the knee inward), thereby reducing the joint load in the knee component.

Studies looking at the benefit of the insoles have been conflicting, as more recent studies have not shown a beneficial effect. Still, it is not unreasonable to try this relatively low-cost and safe treatment.

Bracing

Knee braces are another way to provide stability, support, and pain relief for patients with knee osteoarthritis. There is more than one type of knee brace (a neoprene sleeve versus unloader braces), so your doctor or other health professional, such as an orthotics specialist, can help determine what's appropriate for you. Knee braces should not replace other treatment options, but they can be used along with other treatments. You would need to try using a knee brace to see whether you experience any benefit, and whether your knee feels more stable with less pain.

Occupational therapy

Occupational therapy is all about function—your ability to do things. The goal of occupational therapy is to discover barriers that keep you from functioning normally. Once barriers are identified, the focus switches to finding solutions.

For example, if weakness is identified as a barrier, exercise might be the solution. If walking is a problem, mobility aids may be the solution. Figuring out solutions is necessary so you can remain independent. An occupational therapist can come into your home to evaluate your abilities and level of independence in the kitchen, bathroom, or any other area of your home.

Joint protection and energy conservation

Joint protection can decrease pain and reduce stress on osteoarthritic joints, too, but what, specifically, is joint protection? There are several joint protection principles that, if followed, help to conserve your energy and preserve your joints. The principles focus on proper movement and paying attention to body signals, primarily:

Respect pain
Avoid activities that cause pain (especially if there is
    increased pain the following day)
Use available assistive devices
Use your largest, strongest muscles and joints

Watch your posture and body mechanics

Avoid staying in one position for an extended period

Balance activity and rest

Avoid extended periods with no movement

Lose extra pounds

Pace your activities

Assistive devices for activities of daily living

We mentioned it before: there are many assistive devices available that help compensate for specific limitations. Thirty-five or so years ago, when I was diagnosed with arthritis, these items were hard to find. They are no longer hard to find. There are medical equipment stores near you that carry many of these items. If not, a quick search online is sure to turn up the item you are interested in. There are assistive devices for nearly any activity of daily living.

PHARMACOLOGIC TREATMENT OF OSTEOARTHRITIS

Treating osteoarthritis usually involves medication, whether it is done as self-treatment (using over-the-counter medications) or by going to the doctor to develop a treatment regimen (using prescription medications). Your choices will include over-the-counter acetaminophen (Tylenol), over-the-counter nonsteroidal anti-inflammatory drugs (Aleve, Advil), prescription NSAIDs (ibuprofen, naproxen, Celebrex, meloxicam), and prescription painkillers (hydrocodone, codeine, and tramadol).

All of the aforementioned drugs are commonly used and popular. But which is most effective? Which is safest? A Cochrane review assessed 15 randomized, controlled trials involving 5,986 patients with hip or knee osteoarthritis. For a six-week period, the patients took acetaminophen, NSAIDs, or placebo.

The acetaminophen group had less pain while moving, resting, and sleeping and overall less pain compared with those taking placebo. People who took NSAIDs had less pain and stiffness and better physical function than those who took acetaminophen.

Safety information revealed similarities between acetaminophen and NSAIDs, but study participants taking traditional NSAIDs did have more stomach problems (stomach pain, diarrhea, heartburn, nausea).[7]

NSAIDs are known for their potential adverse effects. Ever since Vioxx was removed from the market in 2004, NSAIDs were labeled with having cardiovascular risks as well as the gastrointestinal risks.

Acetaminophen is known for risk of liver injury, especially if taken with alcohol or overdose or taken at high doses long term. While medications serve a role for controlling pain and inflammation, some patients are turned off by the risks. It's important to weigh risks and benefits when choosing treatments.

Nonoral Topical Medications

Patients who cannot take oral medications have options. There are topical medications such as gels, creams, and patches.

7   T. E. Towheed et al., "Acetaminophen for Osteoarthritis," Cochrane Database of Systematic Reviews 1 (2008), http://www.mrw.interscience.wiley.com/cochrane/clsysrev/articles/CD004257/frame.html.

Some are sold over the counter (capsaicin, Tiger Balm, Bengay), and some are prescription (Voltaren gel and Flector patch).

There is insufficient data to support using rubefacient gels and creams to treat osteoarthritis pain. Rubefacients cause irritation and skin reddening. They are contained in topical products known as counterirritants. They work by offsetting localized pain with local skin irritation.

According to a systematic review by Cochrane researchers, published July 9, 2009, the rubefacient compounds in many topical products are salicylates.[8] Though salicylates are related to aspirin, they don't necessarily work the same when applied to the skin. Topical creams—whether they are counterirritants, salicylates, or capsaicin—are, at best, temporary relief. Topical creams are not intended to be a long-term treatment plan.

Voltaren gel is a prescription nonsteroidal anti-inflammatory drug used to treat pain associated with osteoarthritis in joints that can be managed with topical treatment. Clinical trials demonstrated that Voltaren gel delivers effective pain relief with a favorable safety profile. Its systemic absorption is 94% less than the comparable oral diclofenac treatment.[9] With less systemic absorption, the risk of side effects is less—but there are still the same potential side effects. The Flector patch is a patch that contains diclofenac. The patch can interact

8   P. Matthew et al., "Topical Rubefacients for Acute and Chronic Pain in Adults" (July 2009), http://www2.cochrane.org/reviews/en/ab007403.html.

9   "Voltaren® Gel Receives US Regulatory Approval as the First Approved Topical Prescription Treatment for Pain Associated with Osteoarthritis" (October 22, 2007), http://cws.huginonline.com/N/134323/PR/200710/1161352_5_2.html.

with certain drugs, so be sure to discuss your current drug regimen with your doctor as you consider using the patch.

You're Not Afraid of Needles, Are You?

There are a few treatment options that are given by injection for osteoarthritis. As cartilage wears away in osteoarthritis, synovial fluid changes and becomes a poor lubricant for the affected joint. With a treatment known as **viscosupplementation**, hyaluronan is injected into the knee in an effort to lubricate the affected joint and reduce symptoms. There are several viscosupplements, including Synvisc, Euflexxa, Orthovisc, Monovisc, and Hyalgan. Viscosupplementation has been available to patients since 1997.

Cortisone shots, which were given before viscosupplementation became available, are still a standard treatment offered to patients who have localized pain in a specific joint. Cortisone is a hormone produced in the body. The injections use synthetic cortisone, however. It works by reducing inflammation. Most doctors limit the number of injections you can get per year to three. The fact is that animal studies have shown side effects associated with too many injections, including weakening of tendons and softening of cartilage.

And then there is **acupuncture**. Acupuncture is among the oldest medical procedures in the world, originating in China more than 2,000 years ago. Acupuncture first became well known in the United States in the early 1970s. The acupuncture technique that has been most studied and that most people know as acupuncture involves penetrating the skin with very thin, solid metallic needles that are manipulated by hand or electrical stimulation. Reports suggest that the popularity of acupuncture has grown in the past 10 years. But what you probably really want to know is whether it works. The short answer is there are conflicting reports on its effectiveness. If this interests you, discuss it with your doctor.

THE BOTTOM LINE

The medical management of hip and knee osteoarthritis recommends both nondrug treatments and drug therapy. The guidelines put forth by the American College of Rheumatology are not mandates. The treatment regimen for an individual patient should be decided upon by the patient and his or her doctor. There will be variations between the treatment regimens of different patients.

That's why it's important to give adequate consideration to nondrug treatments, as well as to natural treatments. You owe it to yourself to look beyond traditional medications that are commonly used to control pain. At the very least, nondrug treatments and natural treatments can serve as complementary therapies, to be used *along with* medication, rather than *instead of* medication.

CHAPTER 2

An Overview of Other Types of Arthritis from Dr. Scott Zashin

More than 100 types of arthritis have been identified. Yet the cause of this destructive disorder is still not well understood. Heredity, injury, and/or environmental "insults" are thought to play a role in bringing about the joint destruction that is the hallmark of many types of arthritis. There is no cure for the structural damage from arthritis. For most types of arthritis, treatment is focused on controlling pain and inflammation. The two most prevalent types of arthritis are osteoarthritis and rheumatoid arthritis. You read about osteoarthritis in the previous chapter. Let's now look at rheumatoid arthritis, as well as a few of the other more common types—types you may have heard of.

RHEUMATOID ARTHRITIS: AN AUTOIMMUNE DISORDER THAT AFFECTS THE JOINTS

Rheumatoid arthritis (RA) affects about 1% of the general population. This translates to more than two million Americans, with a 5:2 ratio of women to men. RA strikes many people in the prime of their lives and most often affects people in their early 30s to 60s.

Rheumatoid arthritis is a different illness from osteoarthritis. RA causes considerably more inflammation than osteoarthritis because it is an autoimmune disorder. This means that the body's immune system reacts against itself. In the case of RA, the immune system destroys the joints.

Inflammation results in swelling, warmth, and subsequent pain in the joints. Unlike osteoarthritis, RA affects the entire body. People diagnosed with RA often complain of extreme fatigue and a general sense of malaise.

RA can range in severity from manageable to mildly disabling to completely debilitating. Early diagnosis is important in slowing the progression of joint damage, because damage can sometimes occur in as few as six months of the disease's onset. The challenge, though, is early diagnosis, because RA can be difficult to identify in its initial stages.

Soreness, stiffness, and aching usually begin in the small joints of the feet, wrists, and hands. It is especially common in the knuckles and middle joints of the hands. Pain and inflammation typically occur in the same joints on opposite sides of the body. Morning stiffness usually lasts for 45 minutes or longer, although the stiffness improves throughout the day. Fatigue is common.

RA may affect joints other than the hands, including the feet, knees, elbows, neck, shoulders, hips, and ankles.

Sometimes it affects organ systems such as the lungs or kidneys. Over time, if left untreated, the inflamed joints may become irreversibly damaged and deformed, although this is not always the case.

A doctor can determine whether you have RA based on your symptoms, a physical examination, and results of x-rays and blood tests. Laboratory tests can be very helpful in diagnosing RA. One of the more common diagnostic blood tests for RA screens for a substance in the blood called the rheumatoid factor (RF). Seventy-five percent of patients with RA have this abnormal protein in their blood, although people who do not have RA sometimes have RF in their blood. Some people with RF develop lumps under the skin called rheumatoid nodules. The back of the elbow is a common location. These nodules are usually not painful and typically do not affect joint function.

A newer screening test for RA, called the anti-cyclic citrullinated peptide (CCP) antibody test, was introduced in 2003. This test is considered to be more accurate than screening for RF in patients where RA is suspected. The anti-CCP test screens for the presence of antibodies to CCP (also known as "CCP autoantibodies"). The test has been found to be effective in identifying patients with early, mild arthritis who may be at increased risk for developing a more severe, erosive form of RA.

IS IT OA OR RA?

While osteoarthritis (OA) and rheumatoid arthritis (RA) are the most common types of arthritis, they involve different disease processes. OA is generally described as wear and tear on the joints. RA is a disease associated with an inflammatory process that can cause joint destruction and severe disability. With RA, early diagnosis and aggressive treatment can mean the difference between manageable discomfort and permanent disability.

Osteoarthritis affects the knees and hips, hands and feet, and neck and lower back. RA often begins in the small joints of the hands and feet or knees, and over time larger joints may be affected. The pattern of joint involvement is such that for OA, random joints are affected, but one side of the body may predominate. For RA, there is a symmetric pattern that evolves, with the same joint on opposite sides of the body being affected.

If the hands are involved, OA typically affects the distal finger joints and the basal joint where the thumb connects to the wrist. With RA, the large knuckles (MCP joints) and mid or proximal joints (PIP joints) as well as the wrist is typically involved. There is a difference with morning stiffness, too. With OA, morning stiffness is usually less than 30 minutes in duration but worsens during the day with use. For RA, morning stiffness is prolonged, lasting 45 minutes or longer, and improving as the day goes on.

When RA is suspected, two additional laboratory tests are also usually ordered. The first is the erythrocyte sedimentation rate (ESR) test. The second is the C-reactive protein (CRP) test. Elevated CRP and sedimentation rate are measures of joint inflammation, a key sign of RA.

Like osteoarthritis, there is no cure for rheumatoid arthritis. Treatment focuses on reducing inflammation and preventing further damage, which can help to relieve pain, improve joint mobility, and decrease fatigue. Medications are prescribed to help in these areas and slow the progression of the disease. Diet, exercise, and rest also play a role in improving range of motion, energy, and sense of well-being.

JUVENILE CHRONIC ARTHRITIS

Arthritis can occur in children, and more than 150,000 American youngsters suffer with the disease. The disease has several common names: juvenile arthritis, juvenile rheumatoid arthritis, juvenile idiopathic arthritis, and juvenile chronic arthritis (JCA). Regardless of what it is called, this form of the disease is always defined as arthritis in one or more joints before the age of 16.

Symptoms of juvenile chronic arthritis mimic those seen in adults: pain, stiffness, and swelling in affected joints. Juvenile chronic arthritis may also be accompanied by joint contracture (deformity), joint damage, and changes in growth. Children may also show signs of weakness in their muscles and tenderness in other soft tissues. However, the symptoms may also be elusive, changing from joint to joint and from day to day.

The key sign of juvenile chronic arthritis is symptoms of arthritis in one or more joints that last for six weeks or longer. The child may limp, be reluctant to use a limb, or lack the desire to play and be active. A definitive diagnosis of JCA is based primarily on symptoms, physical examination, and laboratory studies.

Three Types of JCA

While joint inflammation is the common thread in all forms of juvenile chronic arthritis, three patterns of the disease are found among children diagnosed with the disease. Each of these three patterns has different possible outcomes. Therefore, each requires a different approach to treatment.

Pauciarticular onset JCA affects four or fewer joints. It is the most common type of arthritis that affects children. More than half of children with JCA are afflicted with this form of the disease. It affects girls more frequently than boys. Younger children (ages 1 to 5) diagnosed with pauciarticular JCA are at increased risk for inflammatory eye disorders. Regular eye exams are recommended. The antinuclear antibody (ANA) is usually present in blood samples. Pauciarticular JCA in older children is more likely to affect multiple large joints such as the shoulders, hips, and knees.

Systemic onset JCA is the diagnosis for about one or two in 10 children with arthritis. The illness begins with unexplained high fever spikes over 101°F (orally). The fever is often accompanied by a rash that comes and goes. Systemic onset JCA is often associated with an enlarged liver, spleen, and lymph nodes, as well as growth retardation. Arthritis may not develop until several months into the illness. Long-term prognosis is based upon the severity of the arthritis.

Polyarticular JCA affects five or more joints and, often, many more. When laboratory tests are positive for the rheumatoid factor (RF), this pattern of the disease often mimics adult-type RA, with similar symptoms and the risk of progressive joint damage. Children with polyarticular JCA who test negative for RF are less likely to have significant joint involvement and more likely to have a better prognosis.

SPONDYLOARTHROPATHY

Spondyloarthropathy refers to a family of related diseases, including ankylosing spondylitis and psoriatic arthritis. These disorders are characterized by chronic inflammation, especially inflammation of the sacroiliac joints of the spine. Other joints and organs—particularly the eyes, skin, and cardiovascular system—may also be involved.

The spondyloarthropathies share a common genetic marker known as HLA-B27, which can be detected in laboratory tests. Some forms of spondyloarthropathy also share a common pathology called enthesitis. Enthesitis is a chronic inflammation of the site where ligaments and tendons attach to bones.

The most common spondyloarthropathies are:

• Ankylosing spondylitis
• Psoriatic arthritis
• Reactive arthritis
• Inflammatory bowel disease associated with arthritis

There is also a type of spondyloarthropathy called undifferentiated spondyloarthropathy. It has some but not all of the signs and symptoms of one of the specific spondyloarthropathies. Clinical investigators theorize that undifferentiated spondyloarthropathy may simply represent an early phase or incomplete form of ankylosing spondylitis or another spondyloarthropathy. However, clinical study data indicate that undifferentiated spondyloarthropathy may be a distinct form of spondyloarthropathy, just like ankylosing spondylitis, psoriatic arthritis, or reactive arthritis.

ANKYLOSING SPONDYLITI: A RARE ARTHRITIS OF THE SPINE

Ankylosing spondylitis is the most common spondyloarthropathy. The term "ankylosing spondylitis" means, literally, "inflamed spine that fuses together." It is a "seronegative" spondyloarthropathy, meaning that the rheumatoid factor (RF) is not present in the blood of patients with the disorder.

Ankylosing spondylitis affects primarily the spine and sacroiliac joints. The sacroiliac joints are the two joints located at the articulation of the sacrum and the ilium. The ilium is the largest bone of the pelvis. People with ankylosing spondylitis often complain of prolonged morning stiffness in the low back and neck. Ankylosing spondylitis can also cause inflammation of the tendons, eyes, and lungs. Severe cases can lead to fusion of the spine and marked immobility.

Ankylosing spondylitis strikes mostly teenaged males and young adult men. Women who are affected usually have a milder form of the disease. About one in 350,000 Americans has ankylosing spondylitis.

Early diagnosis is important and may help avoid joint damage, deformity, and disability. But diagnosis is often delayed because the symptoms of ankylosing spondylitis mirror that of common back problems. Laboratory tests can aid an accurate diagnosis. Markers for the disease include an elevated sedimentation rate and elevated C-reactive protein, both of which indicate inflammation, as well as a positive HLA-B27 test. Arthritic changes may also be seen on x-rays and in bone scans.

Treatment for ankylosing spondylitis consists of anti-inflammatory medications or TNF blockers, aerobic exercise, and physical therapy. Rehabilitation focuses on proper posture, exercises to strengthen the back and abdomen, breathing exercises to enhance lung capacity, and other exercises to maintain range of motion. Ongoing physical therapy is critical to help avoid a stiff or "ankylosed" spine, which can severely limit mobility and cause permanent disability.

PSORIATIC ARTHRITIS: ARTHRITIS INVOLVING JOINTS AND SKIN

Psoriatic arthritis is an inflammatory condition that is related to the skin condition psoriasis. It is often accompanied by telltale skin patches of raised red areas that have a crusty, silvery scale. The skin lesions usually appear on the scalp, elbows, knees, or lower back, but they may appear anywhere on the body.

About 10% of Americans with psoriasis also have the arthritic form of the disease. Abnormalities of the fingernails and toenails in patients with psoriasis increase the likelihood that they will develop the arthritic form of the disease. Psoriatic arthritis strikes men and women equally and is usually diagnosed between the ages of 30 and 50. Among people who have first-degree relatives (parents and siblings) with psoriatic arthritis, there is an increased risk of developing the disease.

Psoriatic arthritis is a seronegative spondyloarthropathy. It is diagnosed through physical examination, x-rays, and laboratory tests. Lab test abnormalities seen with psoriatic arthritis often mimic RA, except the rheumatoid factor is usually absent and HLA-B27 is present 50% of the time. Psoriatic changes in the skin and nails must also be present before a definitive diagnosis of psoriatic arthritis is made. Treatment focuses on medications to relieve the inflammation, including NSAIDs, Azulfidine (sulfasalazine), methotrexate, and TNF blockers.

Five Patterns of Psoriatic Arthritis

There are five types of psoriatic arthritis. Each is distinguished by the pattern of the involved joints, but all are associated with skin psoriasis.

Symmetric psoriatic arthritis involves pain and swelling in many joints, particularly the small joints of the fingers and toes. It is similar to rheumatoid arthritis in that it affects the same joints on opposite sides of the body.

Asymmetric psoriatic arthritis involves a few joints of the extremities but in a random pattern, such as the fingers on the left hand and toes on the right foot.

Psoriatic spondylitis affects specific joints of the lower spine called the sacroiliac joints. Patients with this type of arthritis typically test positive for the HLA B27 genetic marker.

Distal interphalangeal predominant psoriatic arthritis primarily involves the joints closest to the nails of the fingers and toes. It may also affect other joints. This form of the disease often involves changes in the nails, including pitting, splitting, or degeneration.

Arthritis mutilans is a very rare, painful, and destructive form of psoriatic arthritis that involves inflammation where tendons and ligaments attach to the bone (a condition called enthesitis).

REACTIVE ARTHRITIS

Reactive arthritis is a type of arthritis that occurs in response to an environmental "trigger," such as an infection or injury (thus, the term "reactive"). Like ankylosing spondylitis and psoriatic arthritis, reactive arthritis is a "seronegative" spondyloarthropathy. This means that the rheumatoid factor (RF) is not present in the blood of patients with the disorder.

Reactive arthritis was formerly called Reiter's syndrome. The condition is characterized by inflammation that typically affects three areas: (1) the joints, including the sacroiliac joints of the spine; (2) the urethra, the tube that drains urine from the body; and (3) the eyelids and membranes that cover the eye. (This condition is called conjunctivitis.) A skin rash and inflammation of the mucous membranes, such as the mouth, may also be present.

Symptoms of reactive arthritis usually last for several months to a year. However, symptoms can come and go. In a small number of reactive arthritis patients, the symptoms develop into a chronic form of the disease.

A doctor can determine whether you have reactive arthritis based on your symptoms, medical history, physical examination, and blood tests. Blood tests may be used to rule out other types of arthritis as well as to determine whether a bacterial infection is present. The genetic marker HLA B-27 is found in the blood of a majority of people with this disorder.

X-rays may be ordered to assess the presence of inflammation in the sacroiliac joints of the spine, but x-rays are usually inconclusive in patients in the early stages of reactive arthritis.

Treatment for reactive arthritis includes NSAIDs to relieve inflammation, as well as rest and joint protection. Your physician may also recommend physical therapy or an exercise program to improve mobility of affected joints.

INFLAMMATORY BOWEL DISEASE ASSOCIATED WITH ARTHRITIS

Inflammatory bowel disease (IBD) has two forms: Crohn's disease and ulcerative colitis. Both disorders are thought to be associated with an overactive immune system, which causes inflammation of some portion of the gastrointestinal tract.

About 25% of people diagnosed with IBD also develop arthritis. A small number of patients also develop inflammation of other parts of the body, such as the skin, eyes, or joints. Men and women are affected equally by IBD-associated arthritis, usually between the ages of 25 and 45.

Ulcerative colitis and Crohn's disease have similar signs and symptoms. Diagnosis is aided by physical examination, as well as results of blood tests that confirm the presence of HLA-B27. Treatment for the bowel symptoms depends upon whether the patient has Crohn's disease or ulcerative colitis. Treatment of the underlying bowel disease often helps the arthritis. Other common treatments for the arthritis include injecting the joints with corticosteroids, oral corticosteroids, Azulfidine (sulfasalazine), and tumor necrosis factor (TNF) blockers.

CROHN'S DISEASE

Crohn's disease may cause inflammation of any part of the gastrointestinal tract from the mouth to the rectum, although it usually involves the large intestine (colon) or a portion of the small intestine called the ileum. The inflammation involves all layers of the intestinal wall, which may cause scarring and narrowing of the bowel. Patients with Crohn's disease often complain of symptoms that are similar to ulcerative colitis: fever, weight loss, and loss of appetite. Joint inflammation—particularly of the knees, ankles, and wrists—may also occur, especially at the same time that the bowel symptoms flare. Some patients with Crohn's disease also develop ankylosing spondylitis, which causes back pain.

Crohn's disease is often treated with 5-amino salicylic acid products, such as Azulfidine (sulfasalazine), which helps to control both the bowel symptoms and the arthritis. Corticosteroids and immunosuppressive drugs such as Imuran (azathioprine), as well as the TNF blocker.

Remicade and Humira are alternative drug therapies that can be effective in treating Crohn's disease. In severe cases, surgery may be required to remove the diseased portion of the bowel. While this can eliminate the bothersome bowel symptoms, it may not help with the arthritis, particularly arthritis that affects the spine.

ULCERATIVE COLITIS

Ulcerative colitis causes inflammation and erosion of the lining of the colon. The disease usually begins at the rectum and moves up into the large intestine. Patients with ulcerative colitis often complain of symptoms similar to Crohn's disease: abdominal cramping, fever, and weight loss. Rectal bleeding may also occur. When arthritis is involved, one or more joints may be affected, and the symptoms often move from joint to joint. The most commonly affected joints include the knees and ankles, but any joint may be involved. Unlike RA, involved joints are not typically damaged by the disease process.

As with Crohn's disease, ulcerative colitis is treated with Azulfidine (sulfasalazine), corticosteroids, or immunosuppressive drugs. Surgery can be an effective treatment in severe cases, and unlike Crohn's disease, removal of the diseased portion of the bowel usually eliminates the arthritis.

GOUT: A COMMON AND TREATABLE FORM OF ARTHRITIS

Gout affects more than two million Americans. It is caused by deposits of uric acid, a white odorless crystal that accumulates in the body and causes redness and swelling of the joints.

Attacks come on suddenly and are painful. The big toe, ankle, and knee are common sites of involvement. While gout can occur in men and women of all ages, it rarely occurs in women before menopause.

For a definite diagnosis of gout to be obtained, fluid must be removed from an affected joint and tested for the presence of uric acid. The reason for a joint fluid test rather than a blood test is twofold. First, the uric acid level in the blood may be normal even when gout is present. Second, a high level of uric acid in the blood by itself does not necessarily signify the presence of gout. Nonetheless, the diagnosis can also be made on the basis of clinical features alone.

Medications and diet are often culprits of gout attacks. Certain substances in medications and food can increase levels of uric acid in the blood. Diuretics such as Lasix and hydrochlorothiazide, which are used to treat high blood pressure and edema (fluid retention), can increase the risk of gout attacks. Aspirin also increases uric acid levels and can worsen attacks.

Foods with high purine levels also increase uric acid levels in the blood, so changing your diet may help to prevent attacks. Avoiding sweetbreads, herring, mussels, and sardines can be helpful. So, too, can avoiding alcoholic beverages, especially beer, heavy wines, and champagne. Results of a study published in the *New England Journal of Medicine* indicate that a diet that includes dairy products and vegetables may help to prevent gout. Obesity and overeating or "bingeing" have been associated with gout, so maintaining a reasonable weight may also be a preventative measure.[1]

If frequent gout attacks persist despite changes in medications or diet, your doctor may prescribe certain drugs to prevent flare-ups. These include colchicine, Benemid (probenecid), or Zyloprim (allopurinol).

LUPUS ERYTHEMATOSUS: MARK OF THE WOLF

Lupus erythematosus (pronounced loo-pus air-re-them-atoe-sus) is an autoimmune disorder like RA. The disease was named by clinicians who observed that the skin problems that often signal the condition resembled the facial markings of a wolf ("lupus" means "wolf"; "erythematosus" means "redness").

The cause of lupus is generally unknown. Researchers theorize that the most likely culprit is a genetic disposition toward the disease, combined with a subsequent exposure to some environmental insult or infection that leads to a "confused" immune system that attacks the body's own tissues.

Up to 5% of sisters and daughters of patients with lupus may also develop the disease. It is not uncommon for relatives of lupus patients to have abnormal antibodies in their blood but with no symptoms of the disease. Lower levels of ANAs are often found when RA is also present.

It used to be that only the most severe cases of lupus were diagnosed. Now, due to the sensitivity of newer ANA

---

1   H. K. Choi, K. Atkinson, E. W. Karlson, "Purine-Rich Foods, Dairy and Protein Intake, and the Risk of Gout in Men," *New England Journal of Medicine* 350 (2004): 1093–1103.

blood tests, milder cases of lupus are diagnosed more quickly. Most people with lupus live a normal life with few changes in lifestyle. Nevertheless, detecting the condition early allows patients to be monitored for evidence of more serious illness and treated appropriately.

Treatment of lupus is based on the underlying symptoms. Plaquenil (hydroxychloroquine sulfate), which is also used in RA, may help to control the skin and joint symptoms of lupus, as well as the fatigue. When internal organs such as the kidneys, heart, or lungs are involved, stronger medications may be prescribed. These include Imuran (azathioprine), CellCept (mycophenolate mofetil), or Cytoxan (cyclophosphamide). These medications may be very effective, but they can pose an increased risk of potential side effects.

Some people with lupus do not have to take medications regularly. Prescription drugs (such as corticosteroids) may be ordered as needed for flare-up of symptoms.

Four Types of Lupus

There are four types of lupus. All feature the telltale skin rash that is the hallmark of the disorder. None of the four types of lupus are infectious, nor are they a type of cancer or malignancy. Like RA, people with lupus have an overactive immune system. The number of cases of lupus in the United States is unknown, but experts estimate that up to 1.5 million people may be affected with the disease. Ninety percent of lupus patients are women.

Drug-induced lupus is a rare condition caused from long-term exposure to certain medications. The condition clears up once the offending medication is stopped. However, the presence of ANAs, a marker for lupus, may continue to show in blood tests for a year or more.

Discoid lupus is identified by a skin rash with raised red scaling areas. These lesions sometimes leave scars and are typically seen on the exposed areas. Most people with discoid lupus do not have internal organ involvement, as is seen with the systemic form of the disease.

Subacute lupus, like discoid lupus, is also associated with a skin rash with raised red scaly patches. However, unlike discoid lupus, this form of the disease does not scar.

Systemic lupus erythematosus (SLE). In the 1890s, the famed physician Sir William Osler observed that internal organs—or systems—can also be involved in addition to skin changes associated with lupus. Thus, the term "systemic lupus erythematosus" (SLE) was coined. Symptoms of SLE include arthritis, rash, and flulike symptoms such as aching joints and muscles and fatigue. Infection and sunlight may trigger lupus, but symptoms seem to come and go for no apparent reason. This makes the condition harder to diagnose.

SLE may affect the heart or lungs, where there is usually an inflammation of the organ's lining. This may cause chest pain, especially with breathing. Kidney involvement is not uncommon. Patients may have no symptoms, but a urine test can detect evidence of inflammation. Other systems and regions affected by SLE may include the bone marrow (blood cells), brain, and blood vessels.

Lupus Isn't Always a Clear-Cut Diagnosis

Lupus can be difficult to diagnose. The American College of Rheumatology established 11 criteria to help identify the disorder. A person with lupus usually has four or more of the following symptoms:

1. Malar "butterfly" rash on the cheeks.
2. Discoid skin lesions.
3. Sun sensitivity, where a rash develops from exposure to sun or UV light.
4. Mouth sores, usually on the roof or back of the mouth (typically not painful).
5. Arthritis, with prolonged morning stiffness, usually up to an hour, improving as the day goes on.
6. Abnormal urine test showing large amounts of protein.
7. A history of seizures or psychiatric problems.
8. Sharp pain during breathing due to inflammation of the lining of the lungs or heart, which worsens with deep inhalations (pleurisy).
9. Low white blood count, low platelet count, or evidence of anemia.
10. The presence of antibodies to double-strand DNA (ds-DNA) or of Smith (Sm) antibodies, which are specific for diagnosing lupus.
11. A positive ANA test. Ninety-eight percent of people with lupus have this antibody.

SJOGREN'S SYNDROME: PAINFULLY DRY EYES AND MOUTH

Sjögren's (pronounced show-grens) syndrome is an auto-immune condition. The body's immune system turns against itself, subsequently destroying the exocrine glands that produce tears, saliva, and mucus.

The condition was first described in 1933 by the Swedish physician Henrik Sjögren. He reported women whose arthritis was associated with dryness of their eyes and mouth.

When these symptoms occur without any other rheumatologic condition, it is described as "primary" Sjögren's syndrome. When it occurs with another rheumatologic condition such as lupus, RA, or scleroderma, it is called "secondary" Sjögren's syndrome.

The cause of Sjögren's syndrome is unknown, although scientists believe that genetically predisposed patients may come in contact with a virus or certain bacteria that triggers the immune response. This response inactivates tear and saliva glands. The result is uncomfortably dry eyes and dry mouth.

People with Sjögren's often describe eye irritation and grittiness, as if there is sand in their eyes. A burning sensation in the mouth or throat is also common, as is a hoarse voice or difficulty swallowing, because food sticks to the dry tissue. Enlarged or infected glands that cause pain are also common, as is vaginal dryness among women. Many patients also complain of aching and fatigue.

Sjögren's syndrome affects approximately one in 2,500 people, but the condition is frequently overlooked. A blood test can help to diagnosis the condition. Most people with Sjögren's syndrome have at least one antibody in their blood that is a specific marker for the disease. The markers that may be present in Sjögren's syndrome include:

- Antibodies to the rheumatoid factor (RF), which are found in RA and Sjögren's syndrome
- Those to the ANAs, which are found in RA, Sjögren's syndrome, lupus, and scleroderma
- Those to anti-Sjögren's syndrome A (anti-SSA, or "Ro"), which are found in RA, Sjögren's syndrome, and lupus
- Those to anti-Sjögren's syndrome B (anti-SSB, or "La"), which is diagnostic for primary Sjögren's syndrome

Definitive diagnosis is based on a thorough history and physical examination as well as the results of the laboratory tests to detect the presence of the antibodies that are characteristic of Sjögren's syndrome. A biopsy of the minor salivary gland found in the lips may also be performed.

There is no treatment that is capable of producing normal glandular conditions, so treatment focuses on treating symptoms of dry eyes and mouth. Lubricants, as well as medications that decrease inflammation, stimulate moisture and help patients to feel better.

SCLERODERMA: AN AUTOIMMUNE DISORDER THAT AFFECTS SKIN

Scleroderma is not well understood but is believed to be an autoimmune condition. The term "scleroderma" means, literally, "hard skin," which refers to the smooth, tightened, or thickened areas of skin that are a common sign of the disorder.

Scleroderma is a relatively rare disease. It is estimated that approximately 300,000 Americans have been diagnosed with the disorder. The disease affects all age groups but is most commonly seen in women between the ages of 25 and 55.

Diagnosing scleroderma can be difficult because the symptoms mimic many other diseases. A definite diagnosis is based on a medical history, physical examination, and blood tests. Almost all patients with scleroderma have ANAs in their blood. In addition, a number of scleroderma-specific antibodies may be present in the blood, which can facilitate diagnosis. A skin biopsy can be helpful in diagnosing scleroderma but is not able to differentiate whether the limited or diffuse form of the disease is involved.

There is no cure for scleroderma. Treatment is based on relieving symptoms, particularly those of dry skin and joint inflammation and pain. There are two forms of scleroderma: localized and systemic.

Localized Scleroderma

Localized scleroderma typically affects only a few areas of the skin or several muscles and joints. It is more common in children than adults and rarely develops into the systemic form of the disease. Localized scleroderma is also known as morphea.

Systemic Scleroderma

The second form of scleroderma is called systemic scleroderma. It is also known as systemic sclerosis. This form of the disease involves the skin, as well as the underlying connective tissues, including blood vessels, muscles, bones, and joints. Systemic scleroderma may also affect major organs, such as the heart, lungs, and kidneys.

A diagnosis of systemic scleroderma is usually further classified as one of three types:

Limited scleroderma. This type of systemic scleroderma typically develops slowly over a period of years. It usually affects the skin only on the hands and face. People with limited scleroderma may experience Raynaud's phenomenon (explained below) for years before the thickened, hard skin symptoms characteristic of scleroderma develop.

Limited scleroderma is sometimes called CREST syndrome. The term CREST is an acronym for the five major characteristics of the disorder:

- C—Calcinosis. This refers to the formation of calcium deposits under the skin. These are seen as hard white areas on the skin, usually on the elbows, knees, or fingers. Not all patients with limited scleroderma have calcinosis.
- R—Raynaud's phenomenon. Raynaud's phenomenon is a condition in which the small blood vessels of the fingers or toes narrow in response to cold temperatures

or emotional upset. As the vessels contract, the skin turns white and then blue. As blood flow returns, the skin becomes reddened. Raynaud's (pronounced ray-noze) phenomenon can occasionally damage the tissue, which may result in skin ulcers, scarring, or gangrene.

- E—Esophageal involvement. This is most often described as difficulty in swallowing, due to a poorly functioning muscle in the lower part of the esophagus. This condition can lead to stomach acid backflow into the esophagus, which can cause heartburn, inflammation, and scarring.
- S—Sclerodactyly. This refers to the thickening and tightening of the skin of the fingers, which results in a shiny and slightly puffy appearance. Skin tightening can limit mobility.
- T—Telangietasia. This refers to small areas of redness that most frequently appear on the face, hands, and mouth.

Diffuse scleroderma typically develops over a shorter time frame than the limited type of the disease. The skin symptoms occur quickly and spread over most of the body. Skin thickening may affect the face, chest, and stomach, as well as the upper arms and legs. Like RA, the affected areas are often symmetric. This means that if one side of the body or a limb is involved, the other side is also affected. Diffuse scleroderma may also affect the heart, lungs, or kidneys. Diffuse scleroderma is often cyclical. The disease may be active for several years, followed by a quiet period during which skin symptoms remain stable and joint pain and fatigue lessen.

Sine scleroderma. In recent years, a third type of systemic scleroderma has been identified to describe the form of the disease that causes changes to the internal organs but without hardening or tightening of the skin. This type of systemic sclerosis is called "sine scleroderma." In Latin, "sine" means "without," which refers to the lack of skin involvement in this form of systemic scleroderma.

FIBROMYALGIA: "I HURT ALL OVER"

Fibromyalgia (pronounced fi-bro-my-al-juh) is a very common and often undiagnosed cause of musculoskeletal pain. The condition affects nearly four million Americans, mostly women between the ages of 20 and 50, but it can occur in people of all ages.

People with fibromyalgia typically complain of hurting all over and nonrestful sleep. Even with adequate amounts of sleep, people with fibromyalgia still wake up feeling unrested. The lack of restful sleep seems to exacerbate or worsen the symptoms, resulting in a vicious cycle of increasing fatigue and pain.

There is no laboratory test to diagnose fibromyalgia. It is often a "diagnosis of exclusion," meaning that your doctor will try to rule out other causes of the symptoms. Conditions that must first be ruled out include lupus, rheumatoid arthritis, thyroid disease, and sleep apnea. A diagnosis of fibromyalgia may be confirmed by identifying a number of "tender points," which are certain areas of the body that are painful to the touch.

There is no cure for fibromyalgia, but it is not a deforming or life-threatening disease. The most important aspect of treatment is education. Learning about the condition and what causes the symptoms is very important in recovery. Aerobic exercise for 20 to 30 minutes three or four times a week can also be useful for improving sleep quality.

Many people with rheumatoid arthritis, lupus, and other arthritic conditions may also have fibromyalgia. In fact, fibromyalgia should be considered a possible explanation for symptoms in arthritis patients whose pain is not improving despite improvement in joint swelling.

Chapter 3

The Buzz about Dietary Supplements

Most people know that there are various dietary supplements claiming some level of benefit for joint health, arthritis, and other health concerns. Most also know that dietary supplements are readily available and do not require a prescription from a doctor. But, you need to know even more if you are seriously considering adding dietary supplements to your treatment regimen.

Dietary supplements are a $25-billion industry, according to the *Nutrition Business Journal*.[1] They aren't going away. It's in your best interest to learn about their safe use, whether you decide to use them or not.

WHAT IS A DIETARY SUPPLEMENT?

In 1994, the U.S. Congress defined the term "dietary supplement" in the Dietary Supplement Health and Education Act (DSHEA). A dietary supplement is a product taken by

---

1   NPI Center, "NBJ Reviews the $25 Billion U.S. Supplement Market," *Nutrition Business Journal* (October 15, 2009), http://newhope360.com/diet-products/nbj-reviews-25-billion-us-supplement-market.

mouth that contains a "dietary ingredient" intended to supplement the diet. The "dietary ingredients" in these products may include vitamins, minerals, herbs or other botanicals, amino acids, and substances such as enzymes, organ tissues, glandulars, and metabolites.

Dietary supplements can also be extracts or concentrates and may be found in many forms, such as tablets, capsules, softgels, gelcaps, liquids, and powders. They can also be in other forms, such as a bar, but if they are, information on their label must not represent the product as a conventional food or a sole item of a meal or diet. Whatever their form may be, DSHEA has placed dietary supplements in a special category under the general umbrella of "foods," not drugs, and requires that every supplement be labeled as a dietary supplement.[2]

REGULATORY REQUIREMENTS: ARE THERE ANY?

Before the DSHEA was signed into law by President Clinton, dietary supplements were subject to the same regulatory requirements as other foods. The DSHEA, which amended the Federal Food, Drug, and Cosmetic Act, created a new regulatory framework for the safety and labeling of dietary supplements. It states that a company is responsible for determining that the dietary supplements it manufactures or distributes are safe and that any representations or claims made about them are substantiated by adequate evidence to show that they are not false or misleading.

---

2   National Center for Complementary and Alternative Medicine, "Using Dietary Supplements Wisely" (February 2009), http://nccam.nih.gov/health/supplements/wiseuse.htm.

Dietary supplements do not need approval from the FDA before they are marketed, except in the case of a new dietary ingredient, where premarket review for safety data and other information is required by law. Even so, the manufacturer does not have to provide the FDA with the evidence it relies on to substantiate safety or effectiveness before or after it markets its products.[3]

In 2007, the FDA published guidelines for dietary supplements called Current Good Manufacturing Practices (cGMPs). Consider it a rule book that supplement manufacturers must follow (as of June 2010). Some say it is essential to have cGMPs to ensure high-quality supplements, but others say it doesn't go far enough.

There are also several third-party organizations that offer certification and verification regarding supplement ingredients and quality. Currently, there are four groups offering the third-party verification. You should be aware that they may charge a fee to view their results. United States Pharmacopeia does not charge a fee to see its list of verified supplements (http://www.usp.org/USPVerified/dietarySupplements/supplements.html). ConsumerLab.com, however, requires that you join and become a member to view reports.

- ConsumerLab.com (http://www.consumerlab.com/)
- The Natural Products Association (http://www.npainfo.org/)

---

3   U.S. Food and Drug Administration, "Overview of Dietary Supplements" (October 14, 2009), http://www.fda.gov/Food/DietarySupplements/ConsumerInformation/ucm110417.htm.

- NSF International (http://www.nsf.org/consumer/ dietary_supplements/index.asp?program=DietarySup)
- United States Pharmacopeia (http://www.usp.org/ audiences/consumers/)

What does all of this mean to you? It means that while the manufacturer of a dietary supplement is responsible for ensuring the safety of a product before it is marketed, there is a responsibility that you, as the patient, have to ensure it is safe for you. Look for the symbol on the bottle or supplement package, from one or more of the four authorities listed above, to verify the quality of the product.

WHAT YOU SHOULD DO BEFORE TAKING A DIETARY SUPPLEMENT

If you are considering a dietary supplement, talk to your doctor before using it. Dietary supplements may interact with certain prescription medications or with other dietary supplements. A dietary supplement may also contain ingredients that are not listed on the label. By having a discussion with your doctor about all of the medications and supplements you already use and any you intend to use, you are taking necessary steps to coordinate safe treatment.

THE POPULARITY OF DIETARY SUPPLEMENTS

Using National Health and Nutrition Examination Surveys, researchers evaluated data from two time periods (1988 to 1994 and 2003 to 2006). Between the two time periods, supplement use rose from 42% to 53%. Women were found to be more likely than men to use supplements.

The use of vitamin D and calcium surged during the time frame. Calcium use, among women 60 and older—a group considered at risk for osteoporosis—increased from 28% to 61%. That population of calcium takers would have inadequate calcium levels without supplementation.[4]

In 2007, a national survey found that 17.7% of American adults had used natural products (defined as dietary supplements other than vitamins and minerals) during the previous 12-month period. The most popular products that were used for health reasons during the 30 days prior to the survey included fish oil/omega-3/DHA, echinacea, flaxseed oil or pills, and ginseng, in that order. Another national survey that looked at the use of all dietary supplements found that 52% of adults who responded had used some type of supplement in the 30 days prior to the survey, with multivitamins/minerals, vitamin E, vitamin C, calcium, and B-complex vitamins being the most commonly reported.[2]

HAVE DIETARY SUPPLEMENTS MADE US HEALTHIER?

While supplements may be beneficial for some people, the question has been posed as to whether supplementation is just a replacement for healthy eating. Another interesting fact to consider is that the popularity of dietary supplements has not necessarily translated into improved public health. A researcher from National Sun Yat-Sen University was motivated to study the consequences of health-related

4   J. Gahche et al., "NCHS Data Brief: Dietary Supplement Use among US Adults Has Increased since NHANESIII," *NCHS* 61 (April 2011), http://www.cdc.gov/nchs/data/data-briefs/db61.pdf.

2   National Center for Complementary and Alternative Medicine, "Using Dietary Supplements Wisely" (February 2009), http://nccam.nih.gov/health/supplements/wiseuse.htm.

behaviors among those taking supplements when he observed a colleague choose an unhealthy meal over a healthy meal because he had taken a multivitamin that day. Two experiments were conducted. Study participants were told to take a multivitamin, while participants in the control group were given a placebo. In reality, all of the study participants took a placebo. It was found that those who thought they had taken dietary supplements had less desire to participate in healthy behaviors. In the first experiment, those who thought they had taken a supplement preferred a large buffet meal to a healthy organic meal. In the second experiment, the "supplement takers" walked less to benefit their health than did the control group.[5] Perhaps the biggest boost that comes from dietary supplements is that they make you think that you are doing something to improve your health.

STEERING CLEAR OF FRAUDULENT DIETARY SUPPLEMENTS

The FDA regulators have repeatedly warned us that tainted, dangerous products are marketed as dietary supplements. Some of the products contain hidden prescription drug ingredients at levels that are much higher than what is found in an approved version of the drug. Sound scary? It is. It can be dangerous.

The FDA has received numerous reports of harm caused by these fraudulent products. Most of the fraudulent products promote weight loss, sexual enhancement, or bodybuilding. It's important that you be aware that fraudulent products exist

---

5   "Are Dietary Supplements Working against You?" *Science Daily* (April 21, 2011), http://www.sciencedaily.com/releases/2011/04/110421151923.htm.

and that you be able to identify them and steer clear of them. Here are some warning signs that should make your radar go up regarding a potentially fraudulent or dangerous product:[6]

- Products that claim to be alternatives to prescription drugs.
- Products that claim to have similar effectiveness to prescription drugs.
- Products marketed through mass mailings.
- Products marketed in a foreign language.
- Products that warn that you may test positive in drug tests.

Talk to your doctor. Can't say that enough! Basically, you should ask your doctor whether there are any vitamins and minerals that you need in addition to what you are getting from your diet. If you find any information or marketing materials that seem questionable, take them to your doctor and discuss.

If claims seem too good to be true, take that as a signal that something is awry. Steer clear of buzz words such as "cure" and "completely safe." Also, steer clear of testimonials as the basis for trying a supplement. There is no scientific supporting evidence associated with testimonials. Testimonials are personal experience, not scientific.

REPORTING ADVERSE EFFECTS OF SUPPLEMENTS

If you have used a dietary supplement and experienced a serious side effect, report it. Any adverse effects that you

---

6   "Beware of Fraudulent 'Dietary Supplement'" (March 15, 2011), http://www.fda.gov/ForConsumers/ConsumerUpdates/ucm246744.htm.

believe were directly related to the use of a dietary supplement should be reported to MedWatch. The report can be made by you, your doctor, or anyone with knowledge of the incident by calling the FDA at 1-800-FDA-1088 or faxing at 1-800-FDA-0178. You can also make an online report at https://www.accessdata.fda.gov/scripts/medwatch/medwatch-online.htm.[7]

THE BOTTOM LINE

You can take specific steps to help ensure safe use of dietary supplements. Find quality resources to learn more about supplements. Discuss your intention to use a supplement with your doctor. If your doctor agrees with your intention to try a supplement, stick with the recommended dose. Don't be misled by the term "natural": supplements can cause problems if they interact with what you already take, if they are fraudulent, or if you overdose. Proceed with caution.

QUICK QUIZ: TRUE OR FALSE ABOUT DIETARY SUPPLEMENTS

1. A manufacturer does not have to provide the FDA with the evidence it relies on to substantiate safety or effectiveness before or after it markets its products. TRUE

2. Because dietary supplements are not drugs and do not require a prescription, there is no reason to discuss their use with your doctor. FALSE

3. Dietary supplements may adversely interact with certain prescription medications or with other dietary supplements. TRUE

---

7   "Tips for the Savvy Supplement User: Making Informed Decisions and Evaluating Information" (January 2002), http://www.fda.gov/Food/DietarySupplements/Consumer Information/ucm110567.htm.

4. The FDA regulators have repeatedly warned us that
    tainted, dangerous products are marketed as dietary
    supplements. TRUE

CHAPTER 4
———

The Buzz about CherryFlex

Tart cherries are a delicious nutrient- and antioxidant-rich fruit with potential health benefits. They are marketed as "America's superfruit," distinguishing them from ordinary fruits primarily because of their high levels of antioxidants, pain-relieving benefits, and anti-inflammatory properties.

Red tart cherries have been considered a folk remedy for many years. Substantial anecdotal evidence and personal stories that have been around for decades support the consumption of cherries to relieve arthritis symptoms. But something worth noting has happened with regard to cherries—scientific evidence has begun to catch up.

ARE ALL CHERRIES CREATED EQUAL?

There are more than 1,000 types of cherries grown in 20 different countries around the world. Even with so many varieties of cherries, there are only two main categories of cherries: sweet (also referred to as wild cherries) and sour (also referred to as tart cherries).

It is estimated that 95% of dried, frozen, and juice cherries consumed in the United States are grown on American soil. Michigan, Wisconsin, Utah, Washington, Oregon, Pennsylvania, and New York are among the largest producers of cherries. Michigan alone produces about 75% of each year's cherry crop.

Two major groups of tart cherries exist: morello and amarelle. Morello cherries, such as Balaton, have red pigment in the skin of the fruit as well as throughout the flesh. Amarelle cherries, such as Montmorency, have red pigment in the skin of the fruit, but the flesh of the fruit is clear.

Perhaps this is more than you thought you ever wanted to know about cherries—but you will want to understand their progression from a delicious fruit to an anti-inflammatory agent and antioxidant powerhouse.

WHAT'S IN A CHERRY?

According to the Cherry Marketing Institute, 81% of consumers said they would boost the amount of cherries they eat if they knew the health benefits were essentially those of dietary supplements. So the question becomes: Are they?

NUTRITIONAL VALUE

Tart cherries have been shown to contain similar amounts of antioxidants, if not more, when compared with other berries. The Cherry Marketing Institute indicates that cherries have antioxidant levels comparable to those of blueberries and blackberries but higher than those of raspberries and strawberries.

According to MedlinePlus.com, "Antioxidants are substances that may protect your cells against the effects of free radicals. Free radicals are molecules produced when your body breaks down food, or by environmental exposures like tobacco smoke and radiation. Free radicals can damage cells, and may play a role in heart disease, cancer and other diseases."

Cherries contain anthocyanins (powerful antioxidants that provide the deep red color in cherries), melatonin (an antioxidant thought to improve sleep), and about 17 other antioxidants (including egallic acid, p-coumaric acid, kaempferol, and quercetin), as well as other nutrients (including vitamin A).

AVAILABILITY OF CHERRIES

As you think about adding tart cherries to your diet, consider sources other than just fresh fruit. Cherries are available year-round as dried cherries, frozen cherries, and cherry juice concentrate. Don't know how much you should eat? One serving of cherries is equal to 1/2 cup of dried cherries, 1 cup of frozen cherries, 8 ounces of cherry juice, or 2 tablespoons of cherry juice concentrate. And if you want to bypass all of that, focusing on their nutritional and health impact alone, there is also CherryFlex, a convenient 800-mg softgel capsule and a whole-fruit gel that comes in a jar (http://www. cherryflex.com/).

WHO MAKES CHERRYFLEX?

Cherry Capital Services Inc./Underwood Fruit developed and manufactures the tart cherry paste that is found in numerous CherryFlex products. Founder and co-owner of the company Bob Underwood has spent his 50-year career as a northern Michigan fruit farmer, farm market owner, and nutraceutical/functional food developer.

CherryFlex and a line of other superfruit products are manufactured using a proprietary process with U.S.-grown fruit. The proprietary fruit paste is the only product of its kind made from whole fruit (including skin and pulp). Cherry Capital/Underwood Fruit uses their fruit pastes in softgel capsules, liquid fruit supplements, fruit bars, squeeze pouches, and jars of tart cherry whole-fruit gel. The company is now manufacturing CherryFlex for Dogs and CherryFlex for Horses.

The products are laboratory tested and contain no preservatives, fillers, or additives (http://www.cherryflex.com).

CHERRYFLEX DETAILS

Most antioxidants reside in the skin of fruits or vegetables, so it's significant that CherryFlex utilizes the skin and pulp. In contrast, cherry juice concentrate is made by warming the cherries and pressing them to obtain the juice, while skin and pits are removed and water condensed. Yet another formulation, CherryFlex Liquid, combines the tart cherry paste with cherry juice concentrate.

Analysis

Tart cherries contain flavonoids, chemical compounds that have anti oxidant activity. Anthocyanins (pigment that provides the deep red color of cherries) and quercetin are two types of flavonoids found in cherries and act as potent antioxidants. The certificate of analysis for CherryFlex softgels indicates that there is 112.6 mg of anthocyanins per serving (1 capsule).

CherryFlex has four times the amount of anthocyanins when compared to cherry juice concentrate. The recommended dosage of CherryFlex is one to two softgels per day.

Cost

There are 60 softgel capsules in a bottle of CherryFlex. Depending on how much you take, that could be a one- or two-month supply. The cost is about $21.95 per bottle.

CHERRY RESEARCH

Let's now look to see whether scientific evidence is building and supporting the theory that cherry consumption may help relieve arthritis symptoms through the anti-inflammatory effects of cherries.

University of Michigan Study

Based on a study conducted by the University of Michigan, researchers concluded that a cherry-enriched diet lowered inflammation in animals by 50%.[1] There also have been other studies that suggest anthocyanins in tart cherries may benefit arthritis and other inflammatory conditions.[2] Some studies draw very specific conclusions; for example, studies suggest

---

[1]   "Tart Cherries May Reduce Factors Associated with Heart Disease and Diabetes," University of Michigan (April 2008), http://www2.med.umich.edu/prmc/media/news-room/details.cfm?ID=148.

[2]   "New Studies Link Antioxidant-Rich Tart Cherries to a Healthy Heart," University of Michigan (April 12, 2011), http://www.uofmhealth.org/News/Tart+cherries.

that tart cherries and other antioxidant-rich foods may reduce nitric oxide levels (a compound that has been linked to osteoarthritis and rheumatoid arthritis).[3]

The Winona Study

Two double-blind crossover studies conducted at Winona State University in Winona, Minnesota, examined the effects of CherryFlex supplements on eccentric (eccentric is defined as the lowering phase of exercise such as lowering a dumb bell back down during a biceps curl) exercise-induced inflammation, tissue damage, oxidative stress biomarkers (oxidative stress is defined as a condition when the body's production of free radicals exceeds its ability to neutralize them), and delayed-onset muscle soreness. The results are encouraging: CherryFlex was found to alter muscle soreness following strenuous exercise. From the studies, researchers concluded that taking CherryFlex before or after eccentric exercise may have a protective effect on oxidative stress, inflammation, range of motion, contractile force loss, and perceived pain.[4]

Oregon Health and Science University Study

Study results showed that people who drank tart cherry juice while training for a long-distance run reported significantly less pain after exercise than those who did not drink tart cherry juice. The postexercise benefit can likely be

---

3   "Arthritis/Inflammation/Gout," http://www.choosecherries.com/health/inflammation.aspx.

4   G. M. Kastello et al., "The Effect of Antioxidant CherryFlex Supplementation on Exercise-Induced DOMS, Biomarkers of Tissue Damage, and Oxidative Stress" (November 2008) and "The Effect of CherryFlex Pro Sport Shot Supplementation in Attenuating Eccentric Exercise-Induced Symptoms of DOMS" (November 2010), http://www.brownwoodacres.com/winonastudy.php.

attributed to the anti-inflammatory power of cherries and, specifically, anthocyanins.[5]

Baylor Research Institute

In a 2007 pilot study at the Baylor Research Institute, there were 20 patients in the study who were given a low dose of CherryFlex. More than half of the patients experienced a significant improvement in pain and function after taking the cherry capsules for eight weeks.[6]

Cheribundi for Insomnia

Still another study conducted by researchers from the University of Pennsylvania, University of Rochester, and the VA Center of Canandaigua involved assessing the sleep habits of 15 older adults who drank 8 ounces of tart cherry juice (Cheribundi) in the morning and evening for two weeks and a comparable drink without tart cherry juice for another two weeks. Results showed significant reductions in the severity of insomnia after drinking cherry juice daily.[7]

Cheribundi for Knee Osteoarthritis

Researchers, from the Nicholas Institute of Sports Medicine and Athletic Trauma at Lenox Hill Hospital and the VA Medical Center and University of Pennsylvania,

---

5   K. S. Kuehl et al., "Efficacy of Tart Cherry Juice in Reducing Muscle Pain during Running: A Randomized Controlled Trial," *Journal of the International Society of Sports Nutrition* (May 7, 2010), http://www.jissn.com/content/7/1/17/abstract.

6   Baylor Health Care System, "Can Cherries Relieve the Pain of Osteoarthritis?" *Science Daily* (March 21, 2009), http://www.sciencedaily.com /releases/2009/03/090319164327.htm.

7   W. R. Pigeon, M. Carr, C. Gorman, M. L. Perlis, "Effects of Tart Cherry Juice Beverage on the Sleep of Older Adults with Insomnia: A Pilot Study," *Journal of Medicinal Food* 13 (2010): 579–583, http://sleep.health.am/index.php/sleep/more/tart-cherry-juice-solution-for-insomnia/.

studied the effects of tart cherry juice (Cheribundi) on knee osteoarthritis patients. Their findings were presented at the 2011 American College of Rheumatology Annual Scientific Meeting (abstract no. 1092).

There were 59 patients enrolled in the study. For a 6-week period, 27 of the patients were randomly assigned to drink two 8-ounce bottles of tart cherry juice daily (each containing the equivalent of 45 tart cherries) while the remaining 32 patients were assigned the control (Kool-aid). After one week of not drinking either the cherry juice or the control, the groups switched for another 6 weeks. Results showed that patients drinking the tart cherry juice had less pain based on a standardized measure of osteoarthritis called WOMAC score and significantly less inflammation based on the blood test high-sensitivity CRP (hsCRP).

Some have touted tart cherry juice to help lower uric acid associated with gout. This study did not show any change in uric acid, but also did not study the effect of tart cherries in helping the symptoms of gout. Also of note is that the tart cherry juice was blended with apple juice to decrease tartness. As a result, diabetic patients were excluded from the study because the servings contained 31 grams of sugar.

Dr. Scott J. Zashin's Clinical Experience with CherryFlex

Dr. Zashin has prescribed CherryFlex to more than 300 patients in clinical practice for joint pain and analyzed data for the first 112 patients. Of the participants who had osteoarthritis, fibromyalgia, or rheumatoid arthritis, ultimately 69 qualified to be included in the study and took CherryFlex for three months between October 2005 and November 2007. Three of the original 112 patients were dropped because they had other conditions not covered in the study, 20 subsequently elected not to take CherryFlex, and 20 didn't follow up.

Weight changes, blood pressure, and lab results were monitored to examine possible side effects. Patients were assessed at six weeks and three months. There were six patients who dropped out of the study due to side effects prior to the three-month follow up, but they were included in the results of the study.

Study results concluded that CherryFlex was beneficial and had few side effects. Two patients had lab abnormalities, so the supplement was stopped. One woman in her early 60s was taking four capsules daily instead of the recommended dose of two. There was a slight decline in her hemoglobin (red blood cell count) and a slight decrease in her renal function. Another woman over 65 was taking the product with Celebrex, which is an NSAID and had similar mild blood abnormalities. Both issues resolved within a month of stopping Cherry Flex in this nonpublished, retrospective study (charts were reviewed after the patients took the product). Because I did not re-challenge the women with the product, I cannot say for sure whether or not the supplement was responsible for the lab results.

Due to lack of available data, I do not recommend concentrated cherry products such as Cherry Flex and Cheribundi to my patients who are children, pregnant, attempting to get pregnant or who are breast-feeding.

Dr. Zashin concluded, "Based on my clinical experience, CherryFlex appears safe and well-tolerated. In addition, two CherryFlex capsules contain less than 1 gram of sugar. In my private practice, I have routinely checked the patient's blood (blood count and chemistry) and urine before starting CherryFlex and again within 4 weeks. If the patients elect to remain on the product, I will routinely check their blood work again in 2 to 3 months, then every 4 to 6 months while under my care. While I have not encountered any bleeding issues, I do recommend discontinuation of CherryFlex at least one week prior to elective surgery. As with any over-the-counter product, there are potential side effects, so I would recommend you discuss the use of CherryFlex with your own doctor, especially if you are over 65 years of age, plan to remain on over-the-counter or prescription NSAIDs such as ibuprofen or naproxen, take blood thinners such as Coumadin, Plavix, or other medications that may increase the risk of bleeding. In addition, if you get clinical benefit and plan to take CherryFlex for more than four weeks, it is recommended you follow up with your physician before continuing the treatment."

Double-Blind Placebo-Controlled Study of CherryFlex for Osteoarthritis

A 30-patient double-blind, placebo-controlled study was conducted to further examine the potential benefit of CherryFlex for osteoarthritis. (Research support was provided by Cherry

Capital Services, the manufacturer of CherryFlex). Results from the study failed to show that CherryFlex taken twice daily was more effective than placebo. In essence, the study did not prove that it is effective for osteoarthritis pain. A dramatic, clear-cut response to CherryFlex would have been needed to show efficacy due to the small number of patients enrolled. A much larger study will be needed to prove efficacy, and such a study using higher doses of CherryFlex is currently being considered.

PATIENT STORIES

Some arthritis patients are drawn to natural alternatives, and cherries are no exception. These patients may be fed up with costly prescription drugs or drugs that have undesirable side effects, or they may just be intrigued by "natural." What matters is this: do the natural products work?

In talking to patients who have tried CherryFlex, one thing was abundantly clear: they felt they had nothing to lose by trying it. Most equated "natural" with "safe." Most added CherryFlex to their current treatment regimen aimed at treating various conditions, such as osteoarthritis, fibromyalgia, Sjogren's syndrome, and rheumatoid arthritis. Of those who responded well to CherryFlex, the improvement was apparent in about a month (within a three- to eight-week range).

Matthew C. (fibromyalgia patient)

I was diagnosed with fibromyalgia three years ago. My rheumatologist told me about CherryFlex. I thought it was worth a try, and after just 3 or 4 weeks, I noticed improvement. I had decreased pain.

The fact that CherryFlex is natural was one part of my decision. While I would not have ruled out a prescription medication, the lack of significant side effects and the potential for benefit when combined with the fact that it is natural persuaded me to try it.

I wouldn't say that natural is what I strive for in treatment. However, I will say that I am more comfortable taking a natural product than a prescription drug or most other over-the-counter treatments. If a natural product is generally as effective as some medications, I would definitely prefer to take a natural supplement. What I strive for is relief from symptoms. If that can be achieved in a natural product, I would definitely prefer that option. However, natural products, which are only minimally effective, if at all, would not be something I would consider. In general, I would expect a natural product to be less effective than prescription medications. However, CherryFlex was recommended to me by my doctor with the understanding that the product had been useful in treating symptoms for his other patients. While offering no guarantees, he did stipulate that CherryFlex had relieved some of the symptoms I deal with as a fibromyalgia patient.

I was definitely willing to give CherryFlex a trial run to see if I noticed any difference. However, my expectations for almost every medicine—natural or prescription—are rarely high. This is due to the fact that every medication proves more effective for some people than it does for others. Some medicines, which have been touted as being very beneficial, are not always a good match for me. It is all a matter of trial and error. With each new medication, I am "cautiously optimistic." If it works, all the better. If not, I am less likely to be disappointed from elevated expectations.

CherryFlex was noticeably helpful in alleviating my "background" pain—the day-to-day pain which is noticeable but not excruciating. While it did not prevent or treat "flare-ups," it did allow me to significantly reduce the amount of Aleve and other mild pain relievers I had been taking. I would recommend trying it to anyone looking for an alternative to prescription or over-the-counter pain relievers. My status did not change while taking CherryFlex. I still take neurontin and baclofen. However, I was able to significantly reduce the use of NSAIDs (nonsteroidal anti-inflammatory drugs). Given the possible side effects from moderate NSAID use, CherryFlex was a safe and effective alternative for me. I would especially encourage those who are wary of the risk of bleeding associated with NSAIDs or who are intolerant of some of the pain relievers (aspirin, ibuprofen, naproxen) to try CherryFlex.

Sarah S. (osteoarthritis patient)

I was diagnosed with osteoarthritis about 10 years ago. My hips, spine, hands, and shoulders were painful. I hurt constantly. I had been on prescription meds that were taken off the market. Bextra had helped me so much. I was in so much pain after it was removed. I saw results pretty soon after beginning CherryFlex. I still have some pain but nothing like before. My hands are so much less stiff and less painful. One day I thought, "My hands aren't hurting. I think it must be the CherryFlex."

My doctor recommended CherryFlex to me, and I felt I had nothing to lose by trying. The fact that CherryFlex is a natural product mattered to me. I strive for natural treatment, as much as possible. I am still using CherryFlex, and I believe it is still working. It's all good—nothing bad!

I have not stopped other arthritis medications. I still take Celebrex, arthritis-strength Tylenol, and Ultram, plus the supplement DONA glucosamine.

Kay T. (osteoarthritis, Sjogren's syndrome, Celiac disease)

I have had osteoarthritis for 13 years, Sjogren's syndrome for 24 years, plus celiac for more than nine years. I first heard about CherryFlex from a friend in Houston, and it was also recommended by my doctor a few months later. I began taking CherryFlex in the summer of 2006. Within just a few weeks, I noticed I needed less breakthrough pain medication.

When I was in the hospital for a few days—approximately 6 months after starting CherryFlex—I didn't have any of my supplements with me. I needed MSIR (morphine sulfate immediate-release) to tame the pain. As soon as I was able to go home and get back on CherryFlex, pain subsided within a few days. I also take Medrol, Carlson's fish oil, DONA, and magnesium malate.

I am so glad to find a natural approach that can relieve my pain. Any time that I find a treatment that can reduce the amount of morphine required, well, my body is better for it. It mattered to me that CherryFlex is natural. Though I cannot only use natural products and treatments for arthritis, I like to use as many natural products and treatments as possible.

Sally M. (osteoarthritis)

I was diagnosed with osteoarthritis in 2002. I started using CherryFlex in the fall of 2007. Within two months, I noticed improvement, with less aching in my joints. I have never discontinued the dosage—primarily because I'm feeling too good.

I also take glucosamine, chondroitin, and MSM. I take no prescription medications for my osteoarthritis but do also use Tylenol Arthritis. At one time, I took Celebrex, but since CherryFlex, I have not needed Celebrex.

When CherryFlex was first suggested to me, the fact that it was natural made it an easy decision to try it. I can say two good things about CherryFlex. It's natural! And, it has worked for me!

Debbie B. (osteoarthritis, fibromyalgia, polyarthralgia)

I have been using CherryFlex since January 2007. Two or three weeks after starting CherryFlex, I noticed I was having less joint pain. I had occasion to stop taking it, and the pain returned after one week. I also take AZO cranberry, Citracal, DayPro, and Tylenol. I have not really been able to stop or cut down my other medications or supplements since using CherryFlex.

When CherryFlex was first recommended to me, I didn't just go for it because it was natural. My doctor recommended it, and I trust him completely. I'm not partial to natural treatments—I'm looking for pain relief and whatever helps me achieve it. I'll admit: since CherryFlex is a natural product, my expectations were less than they would have been for a prescription medication, but I felt I had nothing to lose by trying it. I plan to keep taking it—CherryFlex works.

Betty L. (osteoarthritis)

I read about CherryFlex in the Dallas Morning News, *and my doctor also told me about it. I was anxious to try it after hearing about it. I started using CherryFlex in August 2007, and it took about four to six weeks for me to notice any improvement. I noticed that I had less pain when walking.*

I also was taking Tylenol, DONA glucosamine, and hydrocodone. That had been my regular regimen. I quit taking CherryFlex because I became pain free. I currently take no medications.

THE BOTTOM LINE

For decades, on their own, clusters of arthritis sufferers soothed away their pain with tart cherries. By 1950, it was proposed that tart cherries might actually relieve arthritis and gout. Since then, patient experience and scientific evidence have together been building the case for cherries.

For information on how to obtain products mentioned in this book, please go to

www.NaturalArthritisTreatment.com

CHAPTER 5

The Buzz about Glucosamine

The buzz about glucosamine was everywhere back in the 1990s, or so it seemed. As much as we're hearing about vitamin D today, that's what it was then—about glucosamine. Some called it "an arthritis cure" and "a medical miracle." Glucosamine had the potential to halt, reverse, and even possibly cure osteoarthritis, one doctor wrote in a book about the supplement.[1] Those were hefty promises that capture people's attention—and they did.

But over the years, from clinical trials to patient testimonials, the news about glucosamine grew somewhat dimmer. The biggest of the trials was the NIH Glucosamine/Chondroitin Arthritis Intervention Trial, better known as the GAIT trial, but its data weren't published until 2006, years after the hype began. And rather than provide solid conclusions, GAIT even stirred some controversy, as you will see.

---

1   J. Theodakis, MD, *The Arthritis Cure* (New York: St., Martin's Press, 1997; rev. 2003).

GLUCOSAMINE EXPLAINED

Glucosamine is a natural substance that is found in healthy cartilage (the tissue that covers the ends of the bones in joints). More specifically, glucosamine sulfate is a component of glycoaminoglycans, or GAGs, combinations of proteins and sugars that are found in various tissues of the body, including in the matrix of cartilage and in joint fluid.

Studies have shown that taking glucosamine supplements results in pain relief equivalent to some NSAIDs (nonsteroidal anti-inflammatory drugs such as ibuprofen and naproxen). It has also been theorized that glucosamine may slow cartilage damage in osteoarthritis patients.

Glucosamine supplements are derived from the shells of shellfish (e.g., shrimp, lobster, and crab). Glucosamine is available in capsules, tablets, liquid, or a powder that must be mixed with a drink. For any of those formulations, 1,500 mg per day is the recommended dose of glucosamine to treat osteoarthritis.

Many resources suggest that glucosamine should be avoided in patients who are allergic to shellfish, while other resources (including the Arthritis Foundation) recommend talking to your doctor about your known allergy. Most allergies are caused by proteins in shellfish, not by chitin, the substance from which glucosamine is extracted. Again, this is important to discuss with your doctor!

What is clearly emphasized is that if glucosamine has any chance of helping you, it's important to be compliant with the recommended dose. You can stay on your usual arthritis medications while taking glucosamine. If there will be a symptomatic benefit from taking glucosamine, you should notice it within 3 months.

THE SUPPLEMENT INDUSTRY

Since the supplement industry is largely unregulated, you the consumer are left to wonder about the quality and purity of the supplements you purchase. One laboratory (http://www.consumerlab.com) analyzed certain dietary supplements for quality, and it was found that in some cases, the product did not contain the amount of the supplement that was indicated on the label. I don't think any of us believes that paying for an inferior product is acceptable. It is best to stick with large, well-known companies when buying supplements. Reputation is essential when choosing a brand. We'll discuss what many feel is the best glucosamine product in a bit.

POTENTIAL BENEFITS OF GLUCOSAMINE

Primarily, there are three potential benefits of glucosamine. One is that it slows cartilage deterioration. Second, it potentially relieves pain associated with osteoarthritis. Third, glucosamine may improve joint mobility.

RECOMMENDED USE OF GLUCOSAMINE

Knee Osteoarthritis

Based on human clinical trials, there is evidence to support the use of glucosamine sulfate for the treatment of mild to moderate knee osteoarthritis. Most clinical studies have used glucosamine sulfate supplied by one European manufacturer (Rotta Research Laboratorium). It remains unknown whether glucosamine made by other manufacturers is equally effective.[2]

A common criticism of studies that have not found glucosamine to be beneficial is that such studies either included patients with severe osteoarthritis or used products other than glucosamine sulfate. There are other forms of glucosamine, such as glucosamine hydrochloride.[2]

General Osteoarthritis

There have been human clinical studies and animal experiments that offered positive results for glucosamine in treating osteoarthritis of various joints of the body. The evidence is less substantial than what exists for knee osteoarthritis. Pain relief, an anti-inflammatory effect of glucosamine, and improved joint function were among the positive findings. But the studies were deemed not well designed, leaving the door open for more study.

Low-Back Pain

In July 2010, study results were published in the *Journal of the American Medical Association (JAMA)*,[3] focusing on glucosamine as a potential treatment for low-back pain. The

---

2   Mayo Clinic, "Glucosamine Evidence" (updated August 1, 2011), http://www.mayoclinic. com/health/glucosamine/NS_patient-glucosamine/DSECTION=evidence.

3   "Effect of Glucosamine on Pain-Related Disability in Patients with Chronic Low Back Pain and Degenerative Lumbar Osteoarthritis," *JAMA* (July 7, 2010), http://jama.ama-assn.org/ cgi/content/full/304/1/45.

clinical trial was conducted at Oslo University Hospital in Norway and involved 125 patients who took glucosamine sulfate and 125 who took a placebo for six months. Researchers found no significant differences and no reduction in pain-related disability between the glucosamine group and the placebo group, during the study and after one year. The patients involved in this study were older than 25 years old and had lower-back pain for at least six months and degenerative lumbar osteoarthritis.

POSSIBLE SIDE EFFECTS/ADVERSE REACTIONS OF GLUCOSAMINE

There are common side effects associated with glucosamine. Glucosamine may cause mild stomach upset, nausea, heartburn, diarrhea, and constipation and may possibly increase blood glucose, cholesterol, triglycerides, and blood pressure. There have also been reports of glucosamine causing drowsiness, insomnia, headache, skin reactions, sun sensitivity, and nail toughening.[4][5] It is recommended that before stopping the supplement, you should switch brands to see whether the problem resolves. If mild symptoms develop from the product, Dr. Zashin would recommend that his patients discontinue it. Assuming that symptoms improve once off of the supplement, you may consider resuming at a lower dose or trying glucosamine sulfate, if not presently taking this form. You should discontinue glucosamine if side effects recur after changing the dose or the brand.

4   MedlinePlus, "Glucosamine" (August 2009).

5   J. H. Klippel et al., *Primer on the Rheumatic Diseases*, 13th edition (Atlanta, GA: Arthritis Foundation, 2008), 694.

Ultimately, it is not clear whether glucosamine affects blood sugar levels. Some studies have suggested that glucosamine taken by mouth has no effect on blood sugar, while other studies have reported mixed effects on insulin. Caution is advised in patients with diabetes or hypoglycemia and in those taking drugs that are known to affect blood sugar. Caution is also advised in patients with bleeding disorders or those taking drugs that may increase the risk of bleeding. Dosing adjustments may be necessary in such cases.[4] [5]

In women who are pregnant or who are breast-feeding, glucosamine is not recommended due to a lack of scientific evidence pertaining to this population of patients.[4] [5]

THE GAIT TRIALS

The Glucosamine/Chondroitin Arthritis Intervention Trial (GAIT) was a large, randomized, placebo-controlled trial conducted at 16 sites across the United States. In other words, it was the kind of study we are told to pay attention to—those that have a large number of study participants who are randomly assigned the treatment being tested (in this case, glucosamine) or the comparison treatment, which can be a placebo (an inactive substance or dummy pill). Still, in the end, the trial results left questions about the benefits of taking the supplement.

Actually, the GAIT trial was conducted in two parts: a primary study that investigated whether glucosamine, either alone or together with chondroitin, was effective for relieving pain associated with knee osteoarthritis and an additional (ancillary) study that investigated whether glucosamine or chondroitin decreased structural damage associated with knee osteoarthritis.

Primary GAIT 2006

The original GAIT trial was a four-year study to assess the effectiveness of glucosamine. The results were published in the *New England Journal of Medicine* on February 22, 2006. In what came as a surprise to some, study results revealed that the highly touted combination of glucosamine hydrochloride (HCL) and chondroitin sulfate did not provide significant pain relief among all of the study participants. A smaller subgroup of study participants with moderate to severe pain showed significant relief from a combination of the supplements, however.

There were nearly 1,600 study participants with knee osteoarthritis enrolled in GAIT. They were randomly assigned to receive one of five daily treatment courses for 24 weeks:

- Glucosamine HCL alone (1,500 mg)
- Chondroitin sulfate alone (1,200 mg)
- Glucosamine HCL (1,500 mg) and chondroitin sulfate (1,200 mg) in combination
- Placebo
- Celecoxib (200 mg) serving as a positive control

A pain reduction of 20% or more at week 24 compared with pain at the study onset was defined as a positive treatment response. Here's what researchers found:

70% of participants taking Celecoxib experienced 20% or greater pain relief compared with 60% of those taking placebo.

This was considered statistically significant pain relief. But between the other treatments being tested and placebo, there were no significant differences among all participants. Notably, however, 79% of a subgroup of participants with moderate to severe pain experienced a 20% or greater reduction in pain while taking the combination of glucosamine HCL and chondroitin sulfate compared with 54% receiving placebo. Participants in the mild pain subgroup receiving glucosamine and chondroitin sulfate, together or alone, did not experience statistically significant pain relief compared with placebo.[6]

But the relatively small number of participants in the moderate to severe subgroup makes those encouraging results "preliminary," according to rheumatologist Daniel O. Clegg, MD, of the University of Utah School of Medicine, Salt Lake City (lead researcher of GAIT).[7] Of the nearly 1,600 study participants, 78% were in the mild pain subgroup, and 22% were in the moderate to severe pain subgroup.

It should be noted, too, that study participants were allowed to take up to 4,000 mg of acetaminophen daily for pain, except during the 24-hour period before they were assessed at weeks 4, 8, 16, and 24. The use of acetaminophen was reportedly low (averaging fewer than two 500-mg tablets per day). No other NSAIDs (nonsteroidal anti-inflammatory drugs) or opioid analgesics were permitted during the study.

---

6   D. Clegg et al., "Glucosamine, Chondroitin Sulfate, and the Two in Combination for Painful Knee Osteoarthritis," *New England Journal of Medicine* 354 (2006): 795–808, http://www.nejm.org/doi/full/10.1056/NEJMoa052771?siteid=nejm&keytype=ref&ijkey= CWQQcspVDtdCs#t=articleBackground.

7   Efficacy of Glucosamine and Chondroitin Sulfate May Depend on Level of Osteoarthritis Pain, http://nccam.nih.gov/news/2006/022206.htm

Ancillary GAIT 2008

With a subset of participants from the original GAIT study, researchers conducted a two-year ancillary GAIT study at nine sites to assess the prevention of structural damage of joints. Patients from the original GAIT trial were offered the chance to participate in the ancillary study for an additional 18 months—a total of two years. In the ancillary study, the randomly assigned treatments were:

- Glucosamine HCL (500 mg, three times daily)
- Sodium chondroitin sulfate (400 mg, three times daily)
- Combination of glucosamine and chondroitin sulfate
- Placebo
- Celecoxib (200 mg daily)

Enrolled for the ancillary study were 572 GAIT participants with x-ray evidence of moderate to severe knee osteoarthritis in one or both knees.

The results, published in the journal *Arthritis & Rheumatism* in October 2008, revealed that glucosamine and chondroitin sulfate, together or alone, were no more effective than placebo in slowing cartilage loss in knee osteoarthritis (measured as a reduction in joint space width, the distance between the ends of bones in a joint observed on x-ray). But the interpretation of those results was less straightforward than just stated: participants taking placebo had a smaller loss of cartilage than what was predicted. Confusion continued to mount about the effectiveness of glucosamine, and no definite conclusions were drawn.

Two-Year GAIT 2010

While the original and ancillary studies looked at the effectiveness of glucosamine HCL and chondroitin sulfate, taken alone or together, on pain, the two-year GAIT study, published in the *Annals of the Rheumatic Diseases* in June 2010 (http://ard.bmj.com/content/69/8/1459.abstract), evaluated the safety and effectiveness (in terms of pain and function) of the supplements. Participants who took glucosamine and chondroitin, separately or in combination, had outcomes similar to the experiences of patients who took Celebrex or placebo.

In the two-year GAIT, 662 participants were enrolled with moderate to severe knee osteoarthritis. They were randomized to use one of the five treatments in the ancillary study. Researchers concluded that over the two-year period, none of the treatments was clinically different in pain response or function from placebo. Glucosamine and Celecoxib did show "beneficial but not significant trends." Adverse reactions were similar for all treatment groups. Serious adverse events were rare for all treatments.[8]

Dr. Theodakis disputes validity of GAIT

Some people, including Dr. Theodakis (author of *The Arthritis Cure*) had questions—questions about the validity of GAIT. On his own Web site, Dr. Theodakis said, "The study failed. The results shouldn't have even been published. Perhaps this explains the long delay. It appears that the authors manipulated data with a number of statistical adjustments. They refer to this in the article. The study was submitted and subsequently revised."[8]

---

8   "NIH (NIAMS) GAIT (Glucosamine/Chondroitin Arthritis Intervention Trial), Part 2," http://www.drtheo.com/news/documents/documents/Dr.TheosOfficialWebsite-GAIT2.htm.

DONA GLUCOSAMINE

Many doctors recommend DONA glucosamine if you are going to try the supplement. You may be wondering, Why DONA? Quite simply, DONA is the glucosamine sulfate that has been in 90% of clinical trials, and it is the brand with the most clinical evidence for safety and effectiveness. (Recall that glucosamine HCL was used in the disappointing GAIT study). DONA is the trademark name of the original glucosamine sulfate product from Rotta Pharmaceuticals Inc. The recommended dosage and directions from DONA is 2 caplets (750mg each) together daily with water or juice. The product is also available in a powder form.

At the annual meeting of the American College of Rheumatology (ACR) in November 2000, results from a three-year independent clinical trial were presented. The results supported previous study results of DONA glucosamine that concluded it had a positive effect on supporting joint health.

The study reported at ACR in 2000 was conducted in the Prague Institute of Rheumatology and enrolled 202 patients with osteoarthritis who were randomly assigned 1,500 mg glucosamine sulfate once daily or a placebo. The findings verified those reported at the 1999 ACR meeting: glucosamine sulfate significantly decreases progression of knee osteoarthritis over three years.[9] Both studies were carried out according to international guidelines for conducting clinical trials on osteoarthritis drugs.

---

9   "ACR: DONA (Glucosamine Sulfate) Decreases Progression of Knee Osteoarthritis," Doctor's Guide, http://www.pslgroup.com/dg/1E9296.htm.

DONA is sold as a prescription drug in Europe, so it must meet European standards, as do drugs in the United States that are regulated by the U.S. Food and Drug Administration. While DONA is up against tough standards in Europe, you can purchase it off the shelf, without prescription, in the United States. While DONA has been a prescription drug in many countries for a decade, it became available in the United States and Canada in 2001.

Among patients who do well when taking DONA glucosamine, some experience relief from joint stiffness in just two weeks, but the full benefit is realized after about three months.

COCHRANE REVIEW

A Cochrane review, first published in 2001, updated in 2005, and reviewed again in 2008, assessed randomized, controlled trials that evaluated the effectiveness and toxicity of glucosamine as a treatment for osteoarthritis. The update included 25 studies that involved 4,963 osteoarthritis patients. Here's what researchers found:

High-quality studies indicated that pain improved similarly whether the participant was randomized to receive glucosamine or placebo. When all studies were considered (high-quality, low-quality, and old studies), glucosamine improved pain more than placebo.

Studies that tested only the Rotta brand of glucosamine (DONA) showed that glucosamine improved pain more than placebo. This was the case whether the study was high quality, low quality, or old.

High-quality studies showed that DONA glucosamine improved function more than placebo when one type of pain scale was used but not when a different pain scale was used. In terms of safety, side effects affected the same number of participants whether they took glucosamine or placebo. Stomach upset and joint pain appeared to be the main side effects.

The Cochrane review concluded that people with osteoarthritis taking glucosamine may reduce their pain, may improve their physical function, and probably will not experience side effects.[10]

PATIENT STORIES

John A.

I have developed some osteoarthritis in my knee after playing tennis for many years. Tennis is my passion, but the osteoarthritis has all but taken away my ability to play. One of my friends, who also has bad knees, recommended that I try glucosamine. I was reluctant at first but decided there would be no harm in giving it a try. My friend was totally psyched about how much glucosamine has helped him. I'm not one to pill-pop if there isn't a known benefit that's going to come from it, but still, I decided to follow my friend's lead. Unfortunately, that was several months ago, and I

---

10   "Glucosamine Therapy for Treating Osteoarthritis," *Cochrane Review*, http://www2.cochrane.org/reviews/en/ab002946.html.

can't honestly say there has been any change for me. I've now started taking it sporadically rather than as part of a daily regimen, which I doubt is optimal. I feel like I gave it a shot—worth a try—but I'm no glucosamine success story. Probably, I will stop it altogether very soon. I was not taking DONA, however.

Maria H.

My diagnosis is not simply arthritis. My condition is more complex. After having a lumbar/sacral/pelvic x-ray in December 2008 and again in June 2010, it was determined that I have lumbar scoliosis and pelvic torsion. In addition to taking DONA glucosamine, I take a natural anti-inflammatory medication. I believe the combination of both has helped to a degree. It took six weeks of glucosamine before I felt a difference in my joints—less pain and increased flexibility. I took it during the summer months, not the winter, when cold weather is known to bother joints. I also believe my improvement is associated with going to physical therapy. The therapist concluded a tragic fall I had at age 40 jammed my coccyx area up and to the right—and that started musculoskeletal changes and assorted problems. I did have serious problems with constipation while taking DONA.

Sally P.

I have Sjogren's syndrome and fibromyalgia. Also have a problem with aching knees. By word of mouth about 10 years ago, I had heard glucosamine and chondroitin helped aching knees. My doctor suggested that I try glucosamine without chondroitin. I started taking glucosamine about one year ago and saw fast results. My knees no longer hurt at all, and they used to wake me up in the middle of the

night and hurt every morning when I'd wake up. I liked that glucos-
amine was a natural product but would have tried it either way—I
needed something that worked. I tried to keep my treatment regimen
all natural but gave up and also take several medications. My expec-
tations were rather low for glucosamine—I felt I had nothing to lose
by trying it. I still take glucosamine, and it is still working. I have
experienced no negative effects from glucosamine.

THE BOTTOM LINE

Like most treatments, it may or may not help you—and
you won't know unless you try. Some patients swear by it;
others remain dissatisfied. If you are going to try glucosamine,
DONA glucosamine is your best bet, and you should stick with
it for about three months before drawing your own conclusions. Due to the absence of safety data, I do not recommend
glucosamine to my patients who are children, are pregnant or
trying to get pregnant or who are breast-feeding.

CHAPTER 6

—————

The Buzz about Vitamin D

Everyone knows vitamin D is essential for good health—specifically bone health, because it promotes the absorption of calcium. But vitamin D's role is much grander than merely as an ally of calcium. Vitamin D plays a role in the regulation of various genes—perhaps as many as a thousand different genes. Researchers have been studying vitamin D and its connection to specific diseases, looking at how deficiency may increase the risk of certain diseases and how supplementation may help prevent or even treat them.

VITAMIN D EXPLAINED

Calling vitamin D a "vitamin" is somewhat of a misnomer. Vitamins are organic substances that you get from your diet. Vitamin D is produced by your body and is actually a hormone belonging to the group of hormones known as steroids. All hormones in the steroid group are derived from cholesterol. Cortisol, estrogen, progesterone, and testosterone are also in the group. As for vitamin D, there are two forms: vitamin D2 (ergocalciferol) and vitamin D3 (cholecalciferol).

"D" IS THE SUNSHINE VITAMIN

Most people have heard vitamin D referred to as "the sunshine vitamin." When your skin is exposed to UVB (ultraviolet B) radiation from the sun, vitamin D3 is synthesized from a pre–vitamin D molecule, chemically known as 7-dehydrocholesterol. Vitamin D3 is then transported via the bloodstream to the liver, where it becomes 25-hydroxy vitamin D or 25(OH)D, and then to the kidneys, where it becomes 1,25 dihydroxy vitamin D (calcitriol), the biologically active form of vitamin D. From the kidneys, vitamin D travels via the bloodstream to the small intestine, where it participates in the absorption of dietary calcium.

SUN EXPOSURE

Without exposure to UVB, there can be no activated vitamin D. You may think that getting enough vitamin D is a cinch. How hard is it to expose yourself to the sun? But think again: how much time do you really spend in the sun? In our fast-paced, hardworking, computer-driven society, most people do not get nearly enough sun exposure to provide their daily vitamin D requirement. Just 10 to 15 minutes a day is recommended sun exposure to keep vitamin D levels at a sufficient level. But do you get that?

Where you live matters, too. Do you live in a city or town that has 200+ sunny days a year or 200+ cloudy days a year? Even if you do live in a sun-soaked environment, the amount of melanin in your skin makes a difference. Dark African Americans require seven times as much sunlight compared with fair-skinned individuals in order to manufacture their daily requirement of vitamin D. The melanin acts as a natural sunscreen, blocking out the UVB rays needed to make vitamin D.

Even if you were able to bask in the sunshine a lot of the time, there are negative health consequences associated with too much sun exposure. People have been taught to use sunblock products to protect themselves from the harmful effects of the sun. But by blocking the sun, you're blocking the ability to produce vitamin D. Sunscreen with an SPF rating of 15 rating blocks vitamin D production by 99%.[1]

Some folks look to tanning beds as a substitute for natural sunlight. While you may end up with an impressive tan, there are guidelines to follow with indoor tanning. Did you know that the type of lamps used in tanning salons makes a difference? Fluorescent low-pressure tubes emit UVA and UVB rays, whereas round high-pressure lamps emit only UVA. Both UVA and UVB are associated with skin cancer, wrinkles, and an altered immune system.[2]

Are you starting to feel like this is a catch-22? While it's important to understand the connection between the sun and vitamin D, it's essential that you look beyond the sun to harness the benefits of vitamin D.

FOOD SOURCES OF VITAMIN D

Vitamin D can be obtained through food sources and supplements. Eggs, cod liver oil, and fatty fish (e.g., salmon, mackerel,

---

[1]   S. A. Fryhofer, MD, "Vitamin D, Deciphered, Declassified, and Defined for Your Patients," Medscape (March 22, 2010), http://www.medscape.com/viewarticle/718671.

[2]   M. F. Holick, PhD, MD, The Vitamin D Solution (New York: Hudson Street Press, 2010).

and sardines) are excellent sources of vitamin D. Milk and cereals are fortified with vitamin D. Most regular milk is fortified with vitamin D3. Soy milk is typically fortified with vitamin D2. Other dairy products such as yogurt, butter, cottage cheese, and cream are not usually fortified with vitamin D.

You should read labels to be certain of the amount of vitamin D in a particular food product. But diet alone likely won't be enough. A 3.5-ounce serving of salmon, which we just said was an excellent source of vitamin D, offers about 600 IU of vitamin D. An 8-ounce glass of milk provides even less, about 100 IU of vitamin D3. Most people will need to consider supplements to maintain or raise their level of vitamin D.

VITAMIN D SUPPLEMENTS

Vitamins and supplements that are sold over the counter may contain either vitamin D2 or D3. Vitamin D2 is derived from plants and yeast, while vitamin D3 is made from lanolin. According to vitamin D expert Dr. Michael F. Holick,[3] who 40 years ago discovered the active form of vitamin D (1,25 dihydroxy vitamin D), vitamin D2 and vitamin D3 are equally effective in raising blood levels of vitamin D. Another expert, Dr. Sandra A. Fryhofer, suggests that D2 is only one-third as effective as D3 at raising blood levels of vitamin D.

When sold alone and not in combination with another multivitamin or supplement, vitamin D3 is sold in 400 up

---

3   M. F. Holick, MD, "Vitamin D and Chronic Disease Risk" (webinar, December 5, 2008), http://vitamindhealth.org/2009/03/dr-holick%E2%80%99s-responses-to-participant-questions-during-the-december-5-2008-live-webinar-presentation-%E2%80%9Cvitamin-d-chronic-disease-risk%E2%80%9D/.

to 5,000 IU per tablet. There is a higher dose available by prescription: vitamin D2 (brand name Drisdol), a 50,000-IU gelatin capsule or 8,000-IU/mL liquid formulation. Liquid pediatric formulations are also available at 400 IU per drop.

THE ROLE OF VITAMIN D

It is widely known—and has been known for a long time—that vitamin D plays a significant role in regulating calcium and phosphorus levels in the body and in bone growth. Within the past few years, new studies have revealed a broader role for vitamin D in the grand scheme of disease prevention. Vitamin D, it seems, helps to regulate the immune system (by activating T cells), influences genes in charge of cell proliferation, helps to prevent heart disease, and more. There are vitamin D receptors in the many cells of the body, including the brain, prostate, colon, breast, heart, and blood—just to name a few.

Studies have linked vitamin D to lowering the risk of certain diseases such as cancer, heart disease, and autoimmune diseases, including rheumatoid arthritis, lupus, type 1 diabetes, and multiple sclerosis. There's been chatter about vitamin D lowering the risk of osteoporosis, Alzheimer's disease, autism, tuberculosis, and even the flu! The link to osteoporosis is fairly well known. While osteoporosis is most often related to low dietary calcium, insufficient vitamin D also contributes to osteoporosis via reduced calcium absorption, according to the Vitamin D Fact Sheet provided by the NIH (http://ods.od.nih.gov/factsheets/vitamind/).

Experts have suggested that correcting vitamin D deficiency can help relieve symptoms associated with the aforementioned conditions, too—symptoms such as fatigue, joint pain, muscle pain, muscle weakness, chronic pain, headaches, poor memory or concentration, high blood pressure, and bowel or bladder problems. Too good to be true? Perhaps we should temper our enthusiasm just a bit. Remember that only through large-scale, randomized clinical trials can we determine the true benefit of vitamin D, or any supplement for that matter.

In 2010, an analysis of 17 prospective studies and randomized trials concluded that vitamin D supplementation produced a slight but not statistically significant reduction of cardiovascular events. Another review of 13 observational studies and 18 trials showed an insignificant decrease in systolic blood pressure and no change in diastolic blood pressure. In eight of the trials, no effect on glycemia or diabetes was evident. A Cochrane review released in January 2010 concluded that evidence to use vitamin D for chronic pain was poor at present—only one study found a beneficial effect for chronic pain; others found no benefit over placebo.[4]

Let's explain further. An "observational" study is one where researchers compare people with high and low vitamin D levels and correlate their levels with whether they have a disease. The problem therein seems obvious. People with higher vitamin D levels may just have healthier habits than those with low levels. It is "large-scale, randomized clinical trials" that are capable of doling out sturdier conclusions.

---

4   S. Straube et al., "Vitamin D for the Treatment of Chronic Painful Conditions in Adults," Cochrane Database Systematic Review (January 20, 2010), http://www2.cochrane.org/reviews/en/ab007771.html.

Overall, study results related to vitamin D so far—while encouraging in some cases but lacking in others—could even be described as conflicting. As with any good science, it's important to know whether the study design had imperfections. For the layperson, this can be hard to determine; that's why it's important to understand that observational studies don't carry the weight that randomized clinical trials do.

Going all the way back to 1996, in an observational study that looked at a segment of the Framingham study participants (published in the *Annals of Internal Medicine*, September 1, 1996), it was concluded that low intake and serum vitamin D levels were linked with an increased risk for the progression of knee osteoarthritis. In 2009, the Rotterdam study (published in *Journal of Clinical Rheumatology*, August 2009) determined that low vitamin D intake increased the risk of progression of knee osteoarthritis on x-ray, especially among those with low bone mineral density.

Also in 2009, a study was published that considered the effect of serum levels of vitamin D, sun exposure, and cartilage loss from the knee (published in *Arthritis & Rheumatism*, May 2009). There was a correlation drawn, and it was concluded that achieving vitamin D sufficiency may slow cartilage loss in knee osteoarthritis.

Beyond the debate over health benefits of vitamin D, there is also still debate over the levels of deficiency and optimal supplementation.

VITAMIN D LEVELS AND WHAT THEY MEAN

By now, you must be wondering how to determine your vitamin D level and how to know whether it's at a sufficient or deficient level. A simple blood test measures serum levels of 25(OH)D. If the laboratory you use reports separate values for 25(OH)D2 and 25(OH)D3, adding them together gives you the level of 25(OH)D. The value for 25(OH)D2 reflects vitamin D from diet or supplementation, while D3 reflects that obtained through diet, supplements, and sun exposure.

Results can be expressed in nanograms per milliliter or in millimoles per liter. Dr. Sandra A. Fryhofer, in an article for Medscape,[5] states that the consensus for accepted vitamin D levels is:

Vitamin D deficiency: below 20 ng/mL (50 mmol/L)

Vitamin D insufficiency: 21–29 ng/mL (52–72 mmol/L)

Vitamin D sufficiency: 30 ng/mL (75 nmol/L) or more

Vitamin D toxicity: more than 150 ng/mL (374 nmol/L)

Accordingly, up to a billion people in the world, including 30% of Americans, have low vitamin D levels, with as many as 10% of children classified as highly deficient.[5] Some experts believe the optimal level of vitamin D is 40–60 ng/mL. Others suggest that optimal levels of D are 55–90 ng/mL. For reducing the risk of fracture, vitamin D levels must be 40 ng/mL.[6]

---

5   S. A. Fryhofer, MD, "Vitamin D, Deciphered, Declassified, and Defined for Your Patients," Medscape (March 22, 2010), http://www.medscape.com/viewarticle/718671.

6   S. A. Fryhofer, MD, "Vitamin D, Deciphered, Declassified, and Defined for Your Patients," Medscape (March 22, 2010), http://www.medscape.com/viewarticle/718671.

HOW MUCH VITAMIN D SHOULD YOU TAKE TO CORRECT DEFICIENCY?

In general, for every 100 IU of vitamin D consumed, the blood level of 25(OH)D increases by 1 ng/mL. For those found to have a significant deficiency, many doctors prescribe a bolus of 50,000 IU of vitamin D2 once a week for eight to 12 weeks. Beyond that, to maintain a healthy level of vitamin D, there are a couple of options: 50,000 IU of D2 on a regular basis every one to four weeks or daily supplements.

Dr. Holick suggests that 1,000 IU of vitamin D2 or D3 is enough for an individual who is not deficient but strives to maintain vitamin D sufficiency. A double dose (2,000 IU of vitamin D), plus a multivitamin that contains 400 IU of vitamin D, is an appropriate dose for someone who has vitamin D deficiency, according to Dr. Holick.

Healthy people who take a daily dose of 1,000 IU of vitamin D reach their peak vitamin D level in five or six weeks. When vitamin D–deficient patients are treated with 50,000 IU of vitamin D2 once a week for eight weeks, levels begin to increase during the first week of treatment and level off by week 8.[7]

Normal levels may have individual variation based on endogenous production from sun exposure, a person's weight, dietary absorption issues (e.g., people with celiac disease), as well as if someone is supplementing with D2 or D3.

---

7   M. F. Holick, MD, "Vitamin D and Chronic Disease Risk" (webinar, December 5, 2008), http://vitamindhealth.org/2009/03/dr-holick%E2%80%99s-responses-to-participant-questions-during-the-december-5-2008-live-webinar-presentation-%E2%80%9Cvitamin-d-chronic-disease-risk%E2%80%9D/.

HOW TO TAKE VITAMIN D SUPPLEMENTS

Vitamin D supplements can be safely taken with food or milk or on an empty stomach. Time of day is not critical, either. The key is to take an appropriate dose to maintain a sufficient vitamin D level while not taking megadoses that lead to toxicity.

Be sure to check with your doctor before taking vitamin D supplements, especially if you have a medical condition that is associated with elevated levels of calcium (e.g., hyperparathyroidism or kidney stones).

VITAMIN D TOXICITY

There's an expression, "too much of a good thing," and so it is with vitamin D. Too much vitamin D can lead to toxicity. While you can't overdose on vitamin D by spending too much time in the sun or on a tanning bed, you can by taking too much of the supplement.

Vitamin D toxicity is defined as blood levels above 150 ng/mL with high blood calcium, but what you will notice are symptoms associated with toxicity. The symptoms can include nausea, vomiting, loss of appetite, constipation, increased thirst, increased frequency of urination, depression, and weight loss. Serious conditions can develop, including calcification of the kidneys, calcification of major arteries, confusion, and odd behavior.[8]

---

8   M. F. Holick, PhD, MD, The Vitamin D Solution (New York: Hudson Street Press, 2010).

SURGE IN VITAMIN D TESTING

Because of new awareness drawn to vitamin D, doctors have beefed up the testing of their patients. I was diagnosed with rheumatoid arthritis more than 35 years ago, and not until this year did a doctor mention vitamin D or any interest in testing my level. I was initially surprised when my results came back "deficient" but at the same time not surprised after learning more than I ever thought I wanted to know about vitamin D.

A *New York Times* article[9] quotes Quest Diagnostics as having orders for vitamin D tests increase 50% in the fourth quarter of 2009 from the same quarter in 2008. In 2008, a mind-boggling $235 million of vitamin D supplements were bought compared with $40 million in 2001. The numbers have likely spiked again in the year or two since those stats were compiled.

If you don't already have a bottle of vitamin D on hand, you're probably tempted to dash out and get some. After all, no one likes to feel like he or she isn't on the bandwagon. But the overwhelming consensus, if you do your homework, is exactly what we've outlined in this chapter:

- The hype about vitamin D is ahead of the science.
- While study results have been promising, few have come from randomized clinical trials.
- Observational studies can lead to conclusions that are not necessarily cause and effect.

9   T. Parker-Pope, "Vitamin D, Miracle Drug: Is It Science, or Just Talk?" New York Times (February 2, 2010), http://query.nytimes.com/gst/fullpage.html?res=9800EFD8143BF931 A35751C0A9669D8B63.

- There is still debate over optimal levels of D, true health benefits, and concern over high doses.

PATIENT STORIES

From Mary B.:

I was diagnosed in March 2009 with rheumatoid arthritis. I first heard about vitamin D from Dr. Zashin, and after starting a regimen of 50,000 units per week in the spring of 2009, it took seven to eight months to bring my vitamin D level up to the low side of normal. Before that point, I experienced a rapid heart rate.

When vitamin D was recommended to me, I was delighted it was "natural." My expectations regarding natural products are extremely high, and I am trying hard to get healthier and off prescription medications.

My decision to try vitamin D was based on my doctor's recommendation. I am still taking 50,000 units of vitamin D per week and no longer experience a rapid heart rate and generally feel better taking it.

Before starting the vitamin D regimen and arthritis treatment with Dr. Zashin, I had constant pain and an overall feeling of malaise. I simply could not feel comfortable in my own body. With treatment, the overt pain has subsided, and the general feeling of low-grade pain and discomfort has significantly lessened. I continue to take vitamin D because I believe it has helped to make me feel better and because my lab reports show that although my levels have risen, they are still on the low side of normal.

I would encourage anyone to have their vitamin D levels checked. I think the importance of vitamins has generally been overlooked by the medical profession. I am fortunate that Dr. Zashin is one of the enlightened ones. When I first started seeing Dr. Zashin, my labs were pretty dismal, but with treatment, I feel as though I am getting better and feeling stronger every day. It may take a while, but I would prefer a natural approach to better health than prescription drugs.

From Sue M.

My vitamin D level was 6.7 ng/mL in April 2009. I was prescribed 50,000 units once weekly for five months and then switched to 2,000 units of D3 per day. In three months, my vitamin D level normalized, but I was already feeling better, with more energy after just two months!

From Tony G.

I was diagnosed with osteoarthritis in October 2009. I was told by my doctor to take vitamin D after he did a blood test. After two weeks of taking vitamin D supplements, I had noticeable energy, memory, and motivational improvement.

I am taking 5,000 to 10,000 units of vitamin D. I can say this with certainty: life has become more interesting and manageable with normal levels of vitamin D.

MAJOR VITAMIN D STUDY PLANNED

Dr. JoAnn E. Manson, Harvard professor and chief of preventive medicine at Brigham and Women's Hospital in

Boston, is the lead researcher in a major study that will be conducted over the next five years. The nationwide clinical trial, which will be funded by the National Institutes of Health, is recruiting 20,000 older adults, including men 60 years old and older and women 65 and older. The study (http://www.vitalstudy.org) will determine whether high doses of vitamin D and omega-3 fatty acids from fish oil supplements lower heart disease and cancer risk.

THE LATEST NEWS ABOUT VITAMIN D AND RHEUMATIC DISEASE

At EULAR 2010 (the Annual Congress of the European League Against Rheumatism), two separate studies revealed that vitamin D deficiency is common in patients with an array of rheumatic diseases—more than half of whom had lower than normal levels of vitamin D. What was discouraging, however, were reports that supplementation of 800–1,000 IU daily of vitamin D was not enough to bring the majority of rheumatic patients up to sufficient levels. Does this suggest a higher dose would achieve the desired result? That's yet to be determined.

VITAMIN D AND MUSCULOSKELETAL PAIN

Dr. Susan Abou-Raya, a professor of geriatric medicine at the University of Alexandria in Egypt, and colleagues evaluated 265 older patients (age 65 and older) to see whether there was a link between vitamin D status and musculoskeletal pain. In the study, the patients were compared to a control group of 200 patients without musculoskeletal pain. In the group of musculoskeletal pain patients, the mean 25-hydroxy vitamin D level was 18.4 ng/mL compared with 28.9 ng/mL for the control group—a statistically significant difference. Overall, 70% of musculoskeletal patients had suboptimal vitamin D levels compared with 32% of the control group. Approximately 41% of patients with chronic musculoskeletal pain were classified as having vitamin D deficiency compared with a mere 1% of the control group. The researchers concluded that inadequate vitamin D levels should be considered when doctors diagnose musculoskeletal pain conditions.[10]

THE BOTTOM LINE

When it comes to vitamin D's health benefits, we should consider it promising but unproven until larger studies do just that. But there is no downside to reasonably increasing your sun exposure, eating foods rich in vitamin D, and cautious supplementation. Remember, though, that excessive intake of vitamin D supplements can have adverse effects rather than the desired benefits.

---

10   D. Mahoney, "Low Vitamin D Tied to Musculoskeletal Pain," *Rheumatology News* 10 (August 2011): 26, http://www.rheumatologynews.com/article/S1541-9800(11)70522-1/ preview.

CHAPTER 7

The Buzz about ASU
(Avocado Soy Unsaponifiables)

ASU (avocado soybean unsaponifiables), which is classified as a dietary supplement in the United States, hasn't created as much buzz as glucosamine or even vitamin D. But for arthritis patients looking for a natural treatment, ASU may be worthy of consideration. There are a handful of studies that looked at the safety and/or effectiveness of ASU, and the results were promising. Several years ago, ASU was approved in France as a prescription drug. In Denmark, ASU is considered a food supplement.

ASU EXPLAINED

ASU is a natural vegetable extract made from avocado and soybean oils. The unsaponifiable part is isolated from a tiny portion of the oil obtained from avocados and soybeans. To understand "unsaponifiable," you must first understand the meaning of "saponifiable." A saponifiable substance is one that can be mixed with lye to form soap. The oil fractions that are unsaponifiable cannot form soap. They are considered good fats that have health benefits.

POTENTIAL BENEFITS OF ASU

ASU is believed to slow the production of certain inflammatory chemicals in the body and help prevent the breakdown of cartilage. The goal of using ASU is to reduce the need for prescription drugs that may be less safe and have a higher risk for side effects and adverse events.

RECOMMENDED USE OF ASU

The recommended dose of ASU is one 300-mg softgel capsule per day to help minimize the pain and discomfort from osteoarthritis. It may take up to three months to see benefit from taking ASU. The brand Dr. Zashin uses in practice is called AVOSOY.

POSSIBLE SIDE EFFECTS/ADVERSE REACTIONS OF ASU

In controlled clinical studies, ASU exhibited no significant side effects compared with placebo. Mild stomach upset is possible with anything that is ingested, however. It is important to note that ASU has not been studied in children, pregnant women, or women who are nursing.

FOUR PUBLISHED CLINICAL TRIALS FOR ASU

Four high-quality clinical trials were conducted between 1997 and 2002. The conclusions from these studies are the foundation for recommending ASU to osteoarthritis patients.

(1997) Efficacy and safety of ASU in treatment of symptomatic osteoarthritis of knee and hip: a 3-month, randomized, double-blind, placebo-controlled trial

The purpose of this study was to evaluate the effectiveness of ASU in reducing the need for NSAIDs (nonsteroidal anti-inflammatory drugs). Patients with knee or hip osteoarthritis for at least six months and pain for more than three months who required treatment with NSAIDs were given one ASU capsule daily or placebo for three months.

During the initial 45-day period (the first half of the study), patients in both groups were also given one of seven NSAIDs. After day 45, patients were asked to stop the NSAID. During the first half of the study, NSAID use was similar between the ASU and placebo groups. In the second half of the study, an analysis of the number of patients who restarted an NSAID, the mean dosage used, and the time spent off of the drug significantly favored the ASU group rather than the placebo group.

Forty-three patients in the ASU group (56.6%) were able to stay off of NSAIDs throughout the second half of the study compared with only 23 patients in the placebo group (30.3%).

When hip and knee osteoarthritis were considered separately, there were significant reductions in NSAID use in hip osteoarthritis compared with knee osteoarthritis. Among patients with hip osteoarthritis, 21/28 in the ASU group stayed off of NSAIDs—a significantly higher proportion than those taking a placebo. But the difference among knee osteoarthritis patients, 26/48, or 54.2%, in the ASU group was of borderline significance when compared with the placebo group.

Researchers were able to conclude that ASU had a slow-acting effect on symptoms associated with hip and knee osteoarthritis and reduced the need for NSAIDs. ASU was also deemed a well-tolerated treatment.[1]

(1998) Symptomatic efficacy of avocado/soybean unsaponi-fiables in the treatment of osteoarthritis of the knee and hip: a prospective, randomized, double-blind, placebo-controlled, multicenter clinical trial with a six-month treatment period and a two-month followup demonstrating a persistent effect

Another study assessed not only the safety and effectiveness of ASU in the treatment of patients with symptomatic hip and knee osteoarthritis but also the residual effects after stopping treatment. There were 164 patients (114 with knee osteoarthritis and 50 with hip osteoarthritis) in the six-month study that had a two-month posttreatment follow-up period. A 15-day washout period for NSAIDs occurred before the study began so that there was no carryover from the effect of NSAID use. Of the study group, 85 received ASU, and 79 received placebo. At the end of six months, 144 patients were able to be evaluated (75 taking ASU and 69 taking placebo).

Overall functional disability was significantly reduced in the ASU group compared with the placebo group. Pain decreased more in the ASU group compared with placebo. There were fewer patients requiring NSAIDs in the ASU group compared with placebo. Improvement was found to be more significant among patients with hip osteoarthritis versus knee

---

1   F. Blotman et al., "Efficacy and Safety of Avocado/Soybean Unsaponifiables in the Treatment of Symptomatic Osteoarthritis of the Knee and Hip: A Prospective, Multicenter, Three-Month, Randomized, Double-Blind, Placebo-Controlled Trial," *Revue de Rhumatisme (English Edition)* 64 (December 1997): 825–834.

osteoarthritis. There was also found to be a persistent effect from ASU at the end of the two-month follow-up period.[2]

(2001) Symptoms modifying effect of avocado/soybean unsaponifiables (ASU) in knee osteoarthritis: a double-blind, prospective, placebo-controlled study

The effects of 300 or 600 mg of ASU taken daily were compared with placebo in patients with knee osteoarthritis. The study lasted three months and involved male and female knee osteoarthritis patients who were between the age of 45 and 80 years old.

Patients significantly improved with both the 300 and 600 mg doses of ASU compared with placebo. At the end of the three-month study period, 71% of the patients receiving 300 or 600 mg ASU had decreased their use of NSAIDs or analgesics by at least 50%, compared with just 36% of patients receiving placebo. Researchers were able to conclude that ASU at either dosage was more effective than placebo for every endpoint considered. No differences were observed in the effectiveness of the two doses of ASU.[3]

(2002) Structural effect of avocado/soybean unsaponifiables on joint space loss in osteoarthritis of the hip

2   E. Maheu et al., "Symptomatic Efficacy of Avocado/Soybean Unsaponifiables in the Treatment of Osteoarthritis of the Knee and Hip: A Prospective, Randomized, Double-Blind, Placebo-Controlled, Multicenter Clinical Trial with a Six-Month Treatment Period and a Two-Month Followup Demonstrating a Persistent Effect," *Arthritis and Rheumatism* 41 (January 1998): 81–91.

3   T. Appelboom et al., "Symptoms Modifying Effect of Avocado/Soybean Unsaponifiables (ASU) in Knee Osteoarthritis: A Double-blind, Prospective, Placebo-Controlled Study," *Scandinavian Journal of Rheumatology* 30 (2001): 242–247.

The purpose of this two-year study was to evaluate the structural effect of ASU in the treatment of patients with symptomatic hip osteoarthritis. There were 163 patients in the study (102 men and 61 women). The pilot study failed to demonstrate that ASU could have a structural effect on hip osteoarthritis. However, in a subgroup of patients who had advanced joint space narrowing (severe hip osteoarthritis), ASU significantly reduced the progression of joint space loss compared with placebo, suggesting that ASU may have a structural effect. Confirmation of these findings could come if a larger placebo-controlled study in hip osteoarthritis were conducted.[4]

META-ANALYSIS OF ASU STUDIES

Meta-analysis Published in *Osteoarthritis and Cartilage* (2008)

The aforementioned four trials were included in a meta-analysis, in 2008, after a search turned up the small number of controlled, randomized, clinical trials that had evaluated ASU versus placebo to treat osteoarthritis. There were 664 study participants with either knee osteoarthritis (58.6%) or hip osteoarthritis (41.4%) within the four studies.[5]

Researchers concluded from the meta-analysis that there was greater pain reduction with ASU than with placebo. Results led researchers to conclude that a three-month trial

---

4   M. Lequesne et al., "Structural Effect of Avocado/Soybean Unsaponifiables on Joint Space Loss in Osteoarthritis of the Hip," *Arthritis and Rheumatism* 47 (February 2002): 50–58.

5   R. Christensen et al., "Symptomatic Efficacy of Avocado-Soybean Unsponifiables (ASU) in Osteoarthritis Patients: A Meta-Analysis of Randomized Controlled Trials," *Osteoarthritis and Cartilage* 16 (April 2008): 399–408.

of ASU was an appropriate recommendation for osteoarthritis patients. Patients with knee osteoarthritis had a better chance of success with ASU than did hip osteoarthritis patients.[5] ASU has an anti-inflammatory effect that may reduce the breakdown of existing cartilage.[6] Due to the absence of safety data, I do not recommend avocado soy products to my patients who are children, pregnant, attempting to become pregnant or who are breast-feeding.

PATIENT STORIES

Laura L.

I was diagnosed with osteoarthritis about 10 years ago and was treated with Celebrex. My rheumatologist suggested I try avocado-soybean unsaponifiables (ASU). I started taking ASU about 8 or 9 months ago. I would say I felt an improvement after 3–4 weeks. The stiffness I experience on sitting and standing was not as great. I prefer natural remedies at this stage to pharmaceutical remedies with all of their side effects.

I had no expectations when starting ASU. The problem with natural or pharmaceutical medicines is that they work great at first, and then over time their effectiveness decreases. My discomfort is affected by my activity level as well as the bariatric pressure of the weather, so anything that I can take to make me move with greater ease or less discomfort makes my life better. Avocado soy seems to have helped with this, but I didn't know what to expect from it. I felt when my doctor suggested ASU that I had nothing to lose by

---

6   P. Angermann, "Avocado/Soybean Unsaponifiables in the Treatment of Knee and Hip Osteoarthritis," *Ugeskr Laeger* 167 (August 15, 2005): 3023–3025.

trying it. Anything that comes from natural products seems to be less harmful to the body than some of the other medications that I have to take.

I continue to take ASU and Celebrex in combination—but have been able to control my symptoms with just the lowest dose available of Celebrex (100 mg). I feel the combination has helped with the stiffness that I experience with my arthritis. Since I have not stopped taking *ASU, I do not know if my symptoms would be worse without it.*

Gail R.

I was diagnosed with rheumatoid arthritis in 1986. My doctor told me about ASU in late 2009. My husband, who has some degree of osteoarthritis, and I began taking ASU about 9 months ago. I noticed decreased joint and tendon pain about 3 months after starting ASU. My husband also experienced improvement.

My doctor explained that ASU was a natural product with a long track record in Europe. That helped me decide to try it. I have already been on many prescription drugs, and adding a natural product appealed to me. I felt I had nothing to lose by trying it but honestly was skeptical that I would benefit from ASU. My husband and I both still take ASU. I feel less joint pain, especially in my hands. But ASU cannot cure my rheumatoid arthritis, so I take prescription drugs, too. I have experienced no negative side effects from ASU.

THE BOTTOM LINE

If you are looking for the one reason why you should try ASU, it is because the supplement may decrease the pain and discomfort from osteoarthritis. It may also decrease the need for NSAIDs.

Products that say "avocado and/or soy oil" are not the same as ASU. Only about 1% of the oils are the unsaponifiable fraction, and that fraction must be stripped of its nondigestible fiber before active ASU can be absorbed. You can't eat enough avocado or soybean to achieve the same effect.

Remember, the of authors of the respected Cochrane Review of herbal therapy for osteoarthritis concluded, "The evidence for avocado-soybean unsaponifiables in the treatment of osteoarthritis is convincing."[7]

If you want to consider trying ASU, talk to your doctor. Then, choose a reputable manufacturer before you buy ASU. It is best, if tolerated, to stay on ASU for at least three months to determine whether the supplement helps your arthritis.

---

7   Little CV et al. "Herbal Therapy for Treating Osteoarthritis. Cochrane Musculoskeletal Group. July 31, 2000. htttp://onlinelibrary.wiley.com/doi/10.1002/14651858.CD002947/abstract

CHAPTER 8

The Buzz about SAM-e

If you had arthritis in the late 1990s, you probably remember the buzz that surrounded the supplement SAM-e (pronounced Sam-ee). It was touted as an over-the-counter treatment for osteoarthritis and depression, as well as other less prominent ailments. People who were looking for an alternative to what they had been prescribed or those who wanted something natural were eager to learn more about and try SAM-e.

Reports all but offered assurance that SAM-e was safe to use, but its effectiveness was not proven in clinical trials. Still, many people felt they had nothing to lose by trying SAM-e— nothing to lose but the dollars required to buy it, if it turned out not to work.

In 2000, SAM-e was reportedly the twenty-fifth most popular supplement sold in health food stores, and sales were expected to surpass $40 million in 2001. A decade or so later, glucosamine and vitamin D have intercepted the buzz that once surrounded SAM-e. Did it essentially hit a dead end? What happened?

SAM-E EXPLAINED

SAM-e, short for S-adenosyl-L-methionine, is a natural compound found in every cell of the human body. SAM-e is formed in our bodies from methionine (a sulfur-containing amino acid). Amino acids are molecules used to build proteins necessary for your body to function.

THE HISTORY OF SAM-E

The chemical structure of SAM-e was first identified in 1952 by an Italian researcher named Cantoni, 46 years before SAM-e was introduced in the United States as a dietary supplement. When SAM-e was hitting the supplement market in the United States in 1998, it had already been used in Europe for more than a decade to treat osteoarthritis and depression. In Europe, SAM-e is classified as a prescription medication, rather than as a dietary supplement.

Early observations and studies of SAM-e focused on its use for treating depression. Interestingly, some of the clinical trial participants also had osteoarthritis, and they reported that SAM-e seemed to help that condition. Over time, claims surfaced and resurfaced that SAM-e was beneficial for a variety of conditions—but those claims lacked the backing of scientific evidence.

RESEARCH FINDINGS FOR SAM-E

AHRQ Evidence Report (2002)

In 2002, a report about SAM-e was issued by the U.S. Department of Health and Human Services Agency for

Healthcare Research (AHRQ). There were 16 medical professionals who took three years to analyze 102 human clinical trials of SAM-e. Of the 102 studies, 47 were about depression, 14 pertained to osteoarthritis, and 41 of the studies focused on liver disease. These 102 studies were deemed "relevant" following an initial search of 25 databases. The information has now been archived on the AHRQ Web site, and it is considered outdated information, only available for reference purposes.[1]

But what were the highlights of those studies? For osteoarthritis, there was one large clinical trial that yielded a small to moderate effect favoring SAM-e when it was compared with placebo. When SAM-e was compared with NSAIDs (nonsteroidal anti-inflammatory drugs such as ibuprofen, naproxen, and Celebrex), which are regarded as conventional treatment for osteoarthritis, there was no statistically significant difference. In other words, SAM-e was as effective as the standard of care.[1]

BMC Musculoskeletal Disorders: SAM-e versus Celebrex

In 2004, a study was published in *BMC Musculoskeletal Disorders*[2] that compared the effectiveness of SAM-e with celecoxib (better known by its brand name, Celebrex). Celebrex belongs to a newer generation of NSAIDs referred to as COX-2 inhibitors. The study compared a 600-mg dose of SAM-e twice daily with 100 mg celecoxib twice daily for 16 weeks. There

---

1   M. Hardy et al., "S-Adenosyl-L-Methionine for Treatment of Depression, Osteoarthritis, and Liver Disease," Evidence Reports/Technology Assessments, No. 64, *AHRQ* (October 2002), http://www.ncbi.nlm.nih.gov/books/NBK36942.

2   W. I. Najm et al.; "S-Adenosyl methionine (SAMe) versus Celecoxib for the Treatment of Osteoarthritis Symptoms: A Double-Blind Cross-Over Trial," *BMC Musculoskeletal Disorders* 5 (2004): 6. Published February 26, 2004.

were 61 adults diagnosed with knee osteoarthritis enrolled in the study.

The patients were randomly assigned to one of two groups. One group took SAM-e while the other group took celecoxib for the first eight weeks. For the second eight-week phase, the groups switched after a one-week washout period (i.e., they had no arthritis medications for one week). The pills were given according to a double-blind, double-placebo random-ized study design—meaning patients and their doctors did not know what they were taking.

The patients were assessed for pain, improvement of joint function, and side effects for the two treatments. Results indi-cated that SAM-e was equivalent to celecoxib in terms of pain relief and improvement of joint function for osteoarthritis of the knee. SAM-e, though, took about one month to achieve results similar to celecoxib, with the inference being that it took a bit longer than celecoxib.

So, because it took SAM-e longer to start working, COX-2 inhibitors and NSAIDs are said to be more beneficial during the first month of treatment.[2] This finding conflicts with a handful of previous small studies that were only one month in duration but concluded that SAM-e and NSAIDs were equally effective in relieving osteoarthritis symptoms.

The pain-relieving benefit of celecoxib was constant throughout the study, but pain relief from SAM-e increased over time. This led to questions about potential long-term benefits of SAM-e, its effect on progression of osteoarthritis, and whether benefits would have continued after treatment with SAM-e stopped.

Joint function assessments showed steady improvement during the entire study for both SAM-e and celecoxib. Researchers noted that no antidepressive effect was observed in this particular study, so the effectiveness in terms of pain relief and joint function was not due to any antidepressive effect. Some other mode of action was responsible.

With regard to side effects, results of this study agreed with those of previous studies that patients taking SAM-e were less likely to experience side effects compared with patients taking NSAIDs. Overall, SAM-e was considered safe and effective compared with celecoxib, although celecoxib was decidedly better during the first month. When considering results and conclusions, though, we are cautioned to remember that the study had a small number of participants and was not a long-term study.

An interesting side note of this particular study: toward the conclusion of the study, it was determined that SAM-e had lost half of its potency. The study was delayed and a new supply obtained. It was said that this did not affect the study outcomes, but it did bring to mind the importance of quality assurance.

SYNOPSIS OF OLDER SAM-E STUDIES FROM THE 1980S

SAM-e Impact on Hips and Knees

A randomized, double-blind trial verified the effectiveness and tolerance of SAM-e versus ibuprofen in 150 patients with hip and/or knee osteoarthritis. Both SAM-e and ibuprofen were given orally, 400 mg three times daily for 30 days. SAM-e exhibited slightly more effectiveness than ibuprofen for pain management. Minor side effects developed in five patients of the SAM-e group and in 16 patients of the ibuprofen group.[3]

SAM-e versus Ibuprofen

Thirty-six subjects with osteoarthritis of the knee, hip, and/or spine were enrolled in a randomized double-blind study. Patients received SAM-e 1,200 mg daily or 1,200 mg of ibuprofen daily for four weeks. Morning stiffness, pain at rest, pain on motion, crepitus, swelling, and limitation of motion of the affected joints were the parameters considered before and after treatment. There was similar improvement in all parameters in patients treated with SAM-e or ibuprofen, and both SAM-e and ibuprofen were well tolerated.[4]

Clinical Studies: SAM-e and Osteoarthritis

Trials have enrolled about 22,000 patients with osteoarthritis in the past five years, and the consensus supports the effectiveness and tolerability of treatment with SAM-e. This study concluded that the therapeutic activity of SAM-e against osteoarthritis is similar to that of nonsteroidal anti-inflammatory drugs, but the tolerability of SAM-e is higher (meaning patients had less side effects with SAM-e).[5]

---

3   S. Glorioso et al., "SAM-e Impact on Hips and Knees," *International Journal of Clinical Pharmacology Research* (Switzerland) 5 (1985): 39–49.

4   A. Muller-Fassbender et al., "SAMe vs. Ibuprofen," *American Journal of Medicine* 83 (November 20, 1987): 81–83.

5   C. Di Padova, "Clinical Studies: SAME and Osteoarthritis," *American Journal of Medicine* 83 (November 20, 1987): 60–65.

Two-Year Clinical SAM-e Trial on Osteoarthritis

In a longer-term, multicenter, open trial involving 10 general practitioners, the efficacy and tolerance of SAM-e were evaluated for 24 months in 108 patients with knee, hip, and spine osteoarthritis. The patients received 600 mg of SAM-e daily for the first two weeks and 400 mg daily until the end of the twenty-forth month of treatment. Separate evaluations were made for osteoarthritis of the knee, hip, cervical spine, and dorsal/lumbar spine. The severity of symptoms (morning stiffness, pain at rest, and pain on movement) was assessed before the start of the treatment, at the end of the first and second weeks of treatment, and then monthly until the end of the 24-month period. Treatment with SAM-e showed good clinical effectiveness and was well tolerated. The improvement of symptoms with SAM-e was obvious after the first weeks of treatment and continued up to the end of the study. Nonspecific side effects occurred in 20 patients. Most side effects disappeared during the course of therapy. SAM-e administration also improved the depressive feelings sometimes associated with osteoarthritis.[6]

Oral S-adenosylmethionine in primary fibromyalgia

The effectiveness of 800 mg SAM-e daily versus placebo for six weeks was evaluated in 44 patients with primary fibromyalgia. Tender point score, isokinetic muscle strength, disease activity, subjective symptoms (visual analogue scale), mood parameters, and side effects were evaluated. Improvements

---

6   B. Konig, "Two-Year Clinical SAM-e Trial on Osteoarthritis," *American Journal of Medicine* 83 (November 20, 1987): 89–94.

were noted for pain experienced during the last week, fatigue, and morning stiffness in the SAM-e group compared with placebo. The tender point score, isokinetic muscle strength, mood, and side effects did not differ between the SAM-e and placebo groups. SAM-e seemed to offer some beneficial effects for primary fibromyalgia.[7]

WHERE TO PURCHASE SAM-E

SAM-e is available at your local drugstore and general health food store. SAM-e can be found over the counter, in the vitamin and dietary supplement aisle. So, it's not hard to find. What you should do is price comparison—but cheaper is not always better. It's a must to stick with a reputable brand of supplements so you can be assured of quality, even if it does cost a little more. Based on the brand and number of tablets consumed monthly, the cost for SAM-e may be $40 or more per month.

THE BOTTOM LINE

The biggest criticism that you can find about SAM-e is that the supplement doesn't live up to its hype. A similar conclusion was passed down when studies assessed SAM-e for depression. It was found that SAM-e was as effective as prescription antidepressants for easing depression but not more effective.

The Arthritis Foundation has offered some advice on SAM-e. It recommends a dose of 600–1,200 mg daily for osteoarthritis and 1,600 mg daily for depression. But patients are cautioned that SAM-e should not be taken without a doctor's

---

7   S. Jacobsen et al., "Oral S-Adenosylmethionine in Primary Fibromyalgia: Double-Blind Clinical Evaluation," *Scandinavian Journal of Rheumatology* 20 (1991): 294–302.

supervision. Patients are typically advised to take SAM-e with B6, B12, and folic acid supplements. These nutrients are found in a B complex vitamin and help prevent SAM-e from being metabolized into homocysteine, a compound which has been associated with an increased cardiovascular risk. SAM-e may come with the additional supplements included. You should check the label to be sure.[8]

As is the case with most supplements, SAM-e has not been studied by the FDA. Dr. Zashin starts SAM-e patients out at 400 mg and increases every two weeks, if needed for clinical benefit, to a maximum of 400 mg three times a day. Once an effective dose is established, tapering to the lowest effective dose is recommended. It is best to take SAM-e on an empty stomach at least 30 minutes prior to a meal to enhance absorption.

While most studies called SAM-e "tolerable," the Arthritis Foundation reminds us that "high doses of SAM-e can cause flatulence, vomiting, diarrhea, headache and nausea. SAM-e may interact with anti-depressive medications and should be avoided if you have bipolar disorder or are taking monoamine oxidase inhibitors (MAOIs). It may also worsen Parkinson's disease."[9]

SAM-e is not recommended for children, pregnant women or women attempting to become pregnant or who are breast-feeding.

---

8   "PDR for Nutritional Supplements: S-Adenosyl-L- Methionine," *Arthritis Today*, http://www.arthritistoday.org/treatments/supplement- guide/supplements/sam-e.php.

9   "Supplement Guide: SAM-e," *Arthritis Today*, http://www.arthritistoday.org/treatments/supplement-guide/supplements/sam-e.php.

CHAPTER 9

The Buzz about Magnesium

Magnesium is the fourth most abundant mineral in the body. It's essential to good health, playing a role in many normal functions that occur within the body. Yet, magnesium is somewhat overlooked and its significance often understated. Did you know that about 50% of total body magnesium is found in bone? The other half? Just 1% is in the blood, and the remainder is found mostly inside the cells of body tissues and organs.[1]

In part, magnesium is overlooked because people believe the mineral is plentiful in the foods they eat. Mostly, that's true. But keeping an eye on your magnesium level is important. Too little or too much magnesium can wreak havoc.

MAGNESIUM EXPLAINED

Magnesium is required for more than 300 biochemical reactions in the body. Magnesium helps maintain normal muscle

---

1   NIH, ODS, "Dietary Supplement Fact Sheet: Magnesium," http://ods.od.nih.gov/factsheets/magnesium.asp. Accessed August 18, 2010.

and nerve function, maintains steady heart rhythm, supports a healthy immune system, and strengthens teeth and bones. Magnesium also is involved in regulating blood sugar, normal blood pressure, energy metabolism, and protein synthesis[1] The buzz about magnesium comes from the necessity of maintaining adequate body stores of the mineral and its potential role in preventing and managing certain diseases.

MAGNESIUM AND OSTEOPOROSIS

You are aware that calcium and vitamin D are important for bone health. There is also evidence that suggests magnesium deficiency may play a role in postmenopausal osteoporosis—reason being, magnesium deficiency affects calcium metabolism and the hormones that serve to regulate calcium.

Magnesium suppresses the hormone that tells the body to withdraw calcium from the bones, and it stimulates the hormone that tells the body to deposit calcium in your bones. When there is a lack of magnesium, calcium is pulled from the bones, and it can be deposited in soft tissue, causing unwanted medical conditions.

There are no studies to date demonstrating that magnesium supplementation is useful in either preventing bone loss or reducing fracture risk.[2] However, in a study involving older adults, greater magnesium intake was linked to maintaining bone mineral density to a greater level than did lower magnesium intake.[1] More studies are needed to better understand

---

2   International Osteoporosis Foundation, "Other Micronutrients and Bone Health,"http://www.iofbonehealth.org/health-professionals/about-osteoporosis/prevention/nutrition/other-micronutrients-and-bone-health.html. Accessed August 19, 2010.

the role of magnesium in bone metabolism and, consequently, in the development of osteoporosis.

MAGNESIUM AND FIBROMYALGIA

Magnesium as part of a treatment regimen for fibromyalgia came to light after a study was published in the *Journal of Rheumatology* in 1995.[3] The study assessed the safety and effectiveness of Super Malic (a tablet containing 200 mg malic acid and 50 mg magnesium). There were 24 patients with primary fibromyalgia in the study. The study participants were randomly assigned to receive three tablets twice a day in the placebo-controlled four-week trial, which was followed by a six-month open-label dose escalation (patients received up to six tablets twice a day) trial.

Pain and tenderness were the primary outcomes assessed, but function and psychological measures were also considered. Significant reductions in pain and tenderness were seen with dose escalation and a longer treatment period. Researchers concluded that Super Malic was safe and potentially beneficial for fibromyalgia. Other studies have suggested that the combination of calcium and magnesium may be helpful for fibromyalgia patients.

Some researchers believe that fibromyalgia patients have low ATP levels (the energy source for muscles) and that magnesium deficiency makes symptoms worse. Magnesium deficiency also causes an increase in substance P, a body chemical

---

3   "Treatment of Fibromyalgia Syndrome with Super Malic: A Randomized, Double-Blind, Placebo-Controlled, Cross-Over Pilot Study," *Journal of Rheumatology* 22 (May 1995): 953–958, http://www.ncbi.nlm.nih.gov/pubmed/8587088.

responsible for pain perception. Fibromyalgia patients average about three times more substance P than normal.[4]

MAGNESIUM AND MUSCLE CRAMPS

Muscle cramps and spasms can result from magnesium deficiency. Supplementation can help relieve muscle cramps and spasms in such cases. A meta-analysis of 52 randomized trials involving 5,318 patients assessed the incidence of fasciculation (muscular twitching involving the simultaneous contraction of contiguous groups of muscle fibers) and myalgia (pain in the muscles, muscular rheumatism). The incidence of fasciculation was 95% and myalgia was 50% at 24 hours for controls. Muscle relaxants, lidocaine, and magnesium best prevented fasciculation. For myalgia, muscle relaxants, lidocaine, or NSAIDs were deemed the best treatment.[5]

Another study considered the role of magnesium in maintaining muscle integrity and function in older adults. There were 1,453 study participants involved in the InCHIANTI study, which concluded that serum magnesium concentrations were significantly associated with muscle performance, specifically, grip strength, lower-leg muscle power, knee extension torque, and ankle extension strength. Whether magnesium supplements would improve muscle function remains an unknown.[6]

---

4   K. Browning, "The Connection between Magnesium and Fibromyalgia," Associated Content, http://www.associatedcontent.com/article/85339/the_connection_between_magnesium_and.html?cat=5. Accessed August 21, 2010.

5   J. U. Schreiber et al., "Prevention of Succinylcholine-Induced Fasciculation and Myalgia: A Meta-Analysis of Randomized Trials," *Anesthesiology* 103 (October 2005): 877–884, http://www.ncbi.nlm.nih.gov/pubmed/16192781.

6   "Magnesium and Muscle Performance in Older Persons: The InCHIANTI Study," *American Journal of Clinical Nutrition* 84 (August 2006): 419–426, http://www.ajcn.org/cgi/content/abstract/84/2/419/.

MAGNESIUM DEFICIENCY (HYPOMAGNESEMIA)

Magnesium is absorbed in the intestines and transported through the blood to cells and tissues. About one-third to one-half of dietary magnesium is absorbed into the body. While symptoms of magnesium deficiency are rarely seen in the United States, people may not have sufficient body stores of magnesium because of lower than optimal dietary intake.

The level of magnesium in the blood can be too low (hypomagnesemia) because of low dietary intake or malabsorption (when the intestine does not absorb nutrients normally) or when the kidneys excrete too much magnesium. Hypomagnesemia also can be caused by:[7]

- drugs that decrease absorption of nutrients including proton pump inhibitors such as Prilosec, Nexium, Prevacid and Aciphex
- diarrhea
- excessive alcohol consumption
- drugs that increase excretion (including diuretics, antibiotics, some cancer drugs)
- high levels of hormones that increase excretion (aldosteone, antidiuretic hormones, thyroid hormones)
- breast-feeding, which increases magnesium requirements

SYMPTOMS OF MAGNESIUM DEFICIENCY

Symptoms of hypomagnesemia may include nausea, vomiting, loss of appetite, fatigue, and weakness. As magnesium

---

7   "Magnesium" (August 2008), http://www.merckmanuals.com/home/hormonal_and_metabolic_disorders/electrolyte_balance/magnesium.html?qt=&sc=&alt=.

deficiency worsens, numbness, tingling, muscle contractions, muscle cramping, seizures, personality changes, abnormal heart rhythms, and heart spasms can occur. Severe magnesium deficiency can be associated with low blood calcium (hypocalcemia) and low blood potassium (hypokalemia). Obviously, the aforementioned symptoms are also associated with other conditions—that's why an evaluation by a doctor is imperative.

EXCESS MAGNESIUM (HYPERMAGNESEMIA)

The level of magnesium in the blood can be too high (hypermagnesemia). Usually this develops only when people with kidney failure are given magnesium salts or drugs containing magnesium, such as antacids or laxatives.[7] As a result, it is best to avoid taking magnesium if you have kidney disease.

Symptoms of hypermagnesemia include diarrhea, abdominal cramping, weakness, low blood pressure, and impaired breathing—and the heart can even stop beating. Diuretics can increase the excretion of magnesium, but in severe cases, intravenous calcium gluconate, intravenous diuretics, or even dialysis may be required.

RDA (RECOMMENDED DIETARY ALLOWANCE OF MAGNESIUM)

The following recommended dietary allowances for magnesium for children and adults were developed by the Institute of Medicine of the National Academy of Sciences.

Age (Years)	Male (mg/day)	Female (mg/day)	Pregnant (mg/day)	Lactation (mg/day)
1–3	80	80	n/a	n/a
4–8	130	130	n/a	n/a
9–13	240	240	n/a	n/a
14–18	410	360	400	360
19–30	400	310	350	310
31+	420	320	360	320

The recommended adequate intake for magnesium is 30 mg/day for infants 0–6 months old and 75 mg/day for infants 7–12 months old.

FOOD SOURCES OF MAGNESIUM

Green leafy vegetables are rich in magnesium. Unrefined grains and nuts are also high in their magnesium content. Meats and milk have an intermediate level of magnesium content. And, as you might expect, refined foods are typically lowest in magnesium content. Water is variable: hard water has higher magnesium content than soft water.[8] For specific food items, check out the extensive list from the USDA National Nutrient Database: http://www.ars.usda. gov/SP2UserFiles/Place/12354500/Data/SR22/nutrlist/ sr22w304.pdf

Here are some of the foods with the highest magnesium content (taken from the top of that list):

8   L. Pauling, "Food Sources of Magnesium," Institute at Oregon State University (August 2007), http://lpi.oregonstate.edu/infocenter/minerals/magnesium/.

Buckwheat flour, whole groat 301 mg/cup

Snacks, trail mix, regular, with chocolate chips, salted nuts, and seeds 235 mg/cup

Bulgur, dry 230 mg/cup

Oat bran, raw 221 mg/cup

Candies, semisweet chocolate 193 mg/cup

Fish, halibut, Atlantic and Pacific, cooked, dry heat 1/2 fillet 170 mg

Wheat flour, whole grain 166 mg/cup

Spinach, canned, regular pack, drained solids 163 mg/cup

Barley, pearled, raw 158 mg/cup

Spinach, cooked, boiled, drained, without salt 157 mg/cup

Seeds, pumpkin and squash seed kernels, roasted, with salt added 1 oz (142 seeds) 156 mg

Spinach, frozen, chopped or leaf, cooked, boiled, drained, without salt 156 mg/cup

Cornmeal, whole grain, yellow 155 mg/cup

Soybeans, mature cooked, boiled, without salt 148 mg/cup

Snacks, trail mix, tropical 134 mg/cup

Beans, white, mature seeds, canned 134 mg/cup

Beans, black, mature seeds, cooked, boiled, without salt 120 mg/cup

Tomato products, canned, paste, without salt added 110 mg/cup

Cereals ready-to-eat, Kellogg, Kellogg's All-Bran Original 1/2 cup 109 mg

Soybeans, green, cooked, boiled, drained, without salt 108 mg/cup

Fast foods, taco 1 large 108 mg

Nuts, Brazil nuts, dried, unblanched 1 oz (6–8 nuts) 107 mg

Lima beans, immature seeds, frozen, baby, cooked, boiled, drained, without salt 101 mg/cup

Beet greens, cooked, boiled, drained, without salt 98 mg/cup

Beans, navy, mature seeds, cooked, boiled, without salt 96 mg/cup

Refried beans, canned, traditional style (includes USDA commodity) 96 mg/cup

Lima beans, large, mature seeds, canned 94 mg/cup

Okra, frozen, cooked, boiled, drained, without salt 94 mg/cup

Baking chocolate, unsweetened, squares, 1 square 93 mg

Cowpeas, common (black-eyes, crowder, Southern), mature seeds, cooked, boiled, without salt 91 mg/cup

Fish, halibut, Atlantic and Pacific, cooked, dry heat 3 oz 91 mg

MAGNESIUM SUPPLEMENTS

Magnesium supplements are available in different forms, including magnesium malate, magnesium oxide, magnesium gluconate, magnesium chloride, and magnesium citrate salts, plus a number of amino acid chelates (an organic compound combined with metal ions), including magnesium aspartate. Magnesium hydroxide is used as an ingredient in several antacids.

TOXICITY

Toxic effects have not been identified from magnesium ingested from food. But the same can't be said for magnesium supplements. Adverse effects have been seen with supplementation, those we described before as hypermagnesemia. It's extremely important to realize that people with impaired kidney function are the most at-risk group for problems associated with excess supplemental magnesium intake.

POSSIBLE INTERACTIONS

There is the potential for drug interactions with magnesium, so you should be aware of that possibility if you take medications. With antibiotics, magnesium supplements may reduce the absorption of quinolone antibiotics (eg Cipro or Levaquin), tetracycline antibiotics (eg doxycycline and minocycline), and nitrofurantoin. In such cases, it is better to take magnesium one hour before or two hours after taking these antibiotics.[9]

Magnesium may also increase the risk of side effects (dizziness, nausea, and fluid retention) that are associated with calcium channel blockers, including Procardia, Norvasc, Cardizem, Plendil, and Calan. Here are some other concerns:[9]

- Magnesium hydroxide may increase absorption of some drugs used to control blood sugar. The drug you take for blood sugar control may need dose adjustment by your doctor.
- Low levels of magnesium in the blood may increase side effects of digoxin (heart palpitations and nausea). Also, digoxin can cause magnesium to be lost through the urine. Dosage adjustments may be needed.

---

9   "Magnesium," University of Maryland Medical Center, http://www.umm.edu/altmed/articles/magnesium-000313.htm. Accessed August 25, 2010.

- Diuretics may lower magnesium levels, so people on diuretics may be prescribed a magnesium supplement.
- Hormone replacement therapy may help prevent loss of magnesium that occurs during menopause.
- Levothyroxine, a drug used to treat underactive thyroid, may be less effective if magnesium-containing antacids are taken.
- Fosamax and other drugs taken for osteoporosis may have their absorption interfered with by magnesium. Antacids or magnesium should be taken an hour before or two hours after the osteoporosis medications.

There are other drug interactions possible, which is why a doctor should direct your use of magnesium supplements.

DISCUSSION POINTS FOR YOU AND YOUR DOCTOR

Since getting too much or too little magnesium can be a problem, knowing your actual level is important. Talk to your doctor about magnesium. Here are some basic questions that you should discuss.

- Is it likely that I am getting enough magnesium through my diet?
- Is my diet adequate for magnesium intake?
- Should everyone take a magnesium supplement in addition to eating foods rich in magnesium?
- Should I have a blood test to determine my magnesium level and to determine whether I need a magnesium supplement?
- If my blood test comes back within the normal range for magnesium, should I still be retested periodically?

- If my blood test comes back abnormally low for magnesium, should I take a magnesium supplement and should I be retested periodically?
- Could any of my symptoms be linked to my magnesium level?
- What should I consider when choosing a brand of magnesium supplements?

If you elect to have a blood test to determine your magnesium level, Dr. Zashin recommends the "RBC Magnesium" test rather than a magnesium test on blood serum (the fluid portion of blood without cells). The RBC Magnesium test gives you the average of the amount of magnesium that has been in cells in the past four months. The serum magnesium test is a poor indicator since only about 1% of magnesium is stored in blood serum. You may be deficient within your cells but it will not show up in serum for a long time. That's why the RBC Magnesium test is preferred. In patients whose magnesium blood test is not elevated, Dr. Zashin will begin them on one 120 mg Pure Encapsulations brand of magnesium citrate/malate. He typically will increase the dose gradually over one months time if there are no side effects and increased efficacy is needed. He permits his patients to take up to two capsules twice daily.

CHAPTER **10**

The Buzz about Diet and Arthritis

If certain supplements can affect disease symptoms, what about dietary changes? Changing the foods we eat? I don't think anyone considers *diet* an *alternative treatment*. There is no alternative to requiring food, right? But what if *what you eat* or *don't eat* could help control inflammation and arthritis symptoms? If that were proven to be true, I'm sure you would pay attention. I know I would.

A quick search of the Internet turns up many stories from patients who claim that changing their diet helped arthritis symptoms. But, is there scientific evidence to back up the positive patient stories about diet and arthritis?

DIET ADVICE

There's no shortage of "advice" about diet and arthritis available. The problem is figuring out how to differentiate sound advice from useless advice. Since there are different types of arthritis, how can you tell whether a discussion about diet and arthritis applies to your type of arthritis or whether there is even a glimmer of benefit that can be derived from suggested dietary changes?

The best advice, when it comes to diet and arthritis, is to keep your expectations realistic. There is no scientific evidence that *proves* what you eat causes or *cures* arthritis, the exception being gout, which is linked to diet.[1]

There is a growing body of scientific literature, though, that suggests dietary changes may relieve arthritis symptoms. Mostly, that literature pertains to the anti-inflammatory effects of certain foods. Logically speaking, an anti-inflammatory diet would mostly impact inflammatory types of arthritis, such as rheumatoid arthritis and psoriatic arthritis. Osteoarthritis is not classified as an inflammatory arthritis, but researchers believe that inflammation plays some role in osteoarthritis. According to researchers, MRIs taken during the early stages of osteoarthritis sometimes detect synovitis (inflammation of joint lining) even though the joint cartilage still appears normal. This might suggest that other joint structures are involved in triggering inflammation in osteoarthritis.

DIET AND OSTEOARTHRITIS

Let's look at some of the available scientific evidence. In one study, published in *BioMed Central Musculoskeletal Disorders*, researchers from King's College in London analyzed the diets and x-ray findings of 1,000 women.

---

1   "Dietary Garlic and Hip Osteoarthritis: Evidence of a Protective Effect and Putative Mechanism of Action," *BMC Musculoskeletal Disorders* 11 (2010): 280, doi:10.1186/1471-2474-11-280, http://www.biomedcentral.com/1471-2474/11/280/abstract.

There appeared to be less early evidence of hip osteoarthritis among the women who ate a substantial amount of fruits and vegetables, especially garlic, onions, leeks, chives, scallions, and other vegetables in the "allium" family. Allium is a genus of plants with 500 species. Allium plants, which are of the lily family, grow from bulbs.

Researchers also found, in a laboratory setting, that a compound in garlic (diallyl disulphide) limited cartilage-damaging enzymes in human cells. While that sounds like a significant finding, researchers did not advise patients to add garlic to their meals or gobble up garlic supplements.[1]

Another study, in the United Kingdom, concluded that sulforaphane, a compound found in broccoli, may prevent the breakdown of cartilage by blocking enzymes that play a role in cartilage degradation. The professor from East Anglia's School of Biological Sciences pointed out that there is still much to be proven or disproven regarding the beneficial effect of broccoli, but at this point, you can't go wrong: broccoli is healthful and is high in fiber and antioxidants.[2]

DIET AND RHEUMATOID ARTHRITIS

In 2008, an analysis of studies relevant to dietary intervention and rheumatoid arthritis was published in the respected Cochrane review. There were 15 studies ultimately selected that involved 837 patients. Researchers concluded that the effect of dietary changes on rheumatoid arthritis—whether a

---

2 "Eating Broccoli Could Guard against Arthritis," University of East Anglia's School of Biological Sciences (September 2010), http://www.uea.ac.uk/bio/news/broccoli.

vegetarian diet, a Mediterranean diet, or an elimination diet—is uncertain. The studies in the review were small, and there was some degree of bias.

Also, it was pointed out that patients on diets may consequentially lose weight, whether they planned to or not.[3] That would be viewed as a positive consequence if you were overweight or a negative if you were underweight. Beyond that, researchers concluded that another negative issue is that diets are hard to stick to, resulting in noncompliance and a high dropout rate.

ANTI-INFLAMMATORY DIET

The key to an anti-inflammatory diet is to avoid foods that promote inflammation and eat a diet that is rich in anti-inflammatory foods. That's the premise: certain foods increase inflammation, while other foods decrease inflammation.

Researchers know that certain enzymes (COX-1 and COX-2) are involved with inflammation. COX-2 enzymes cause increased inflammation when you ingest more omega-6 fatty acids than omega-3 fatty acids. Omega-3 and omega-6 fatty acids are referred to as "essential fatty acids." What that means is that the essential fatty acids must come to us through our diet. The body does not manufacture essential fatty acids on its own.

Omega-3 and omega-6 fatty acids are also involved in building hormones, but those hormones have opposite effects. Hormones built with omega-6 fatty acids promote

---

3   "Dietary Interventions for Rheumatoid Arthritis," Cochrane Library (September 2009), http://onlinelibrary.wiley.com/doi/10.1002/14651858.CD006400.pub2/abstract.

inflammation, while those built with omega-3 fatty acids decrease inflammation.

Omega-3 and omega-6 fatty acids are polyunsaturated fatty acids (PUFA). Their chemical structure differs a bit, and how they work in our body differs. It's important to know which foods are high in omega-3 fatty acids and which are high in omega-6 fatty acids.

There are few food sources of omega-3 fatty acids. Primarily, omega-3 fatty acids come from the fat of cold-water fish (salmon, sardines, herring, mackerel, black cod, and blue-fish). Omega-6 fatty acids, on the other hand, are found in seeds and nuts and the oils derived from them. That means we get omega-6 fatty acids in snack foods, as well as fried foods, egg yolks, and meats—generally, what we consider to be junk food or fatty foods.[4]

Not all nuts are equal. Some have a better ratio than others. For example, walnuts contain a precursor omega-3, known as alpha-linolenic acid, or ALA. Walnuts also contain the highest amount of omega-3-fatty acids in 1 ounce of nuts compared with other nuts (2.5 g of omega-3 fatty acids versus less than 0.5 g found in other nuts).[5] In terms of omega-6 levels, walnuts have 10.8 g in 1 ounce, whereas almonds have 3.5 g of omega-6 fatty acids in an ounce.[6]

---

4   A. Weil, "Balancing Omega 3 and Omega 6" (February 22, 2007), http://www.drweil.com/drw/u/QAA400149/balancing-omega-3-and-omega-6.html.

5   J. Moll, "The Walnut: One of the Heart Friendly, Healthy Nuts" (January 21, 2011), http://cholesterol.about.com/od/treatments/a/walnut.htm.

6   "Omega-3 Fatty Acids," Tufts University, http://ocw.tufts.edu/data/47/531409.pdf. Accessed September 4, 2011.

At one time, people consumed a diet that kept omega-3 fatty acids and omega-6 fatty acids in balance, but that is no longer the case for many people. Too many of us rely heavily on processed foods and fast food. While both omega-3s and omega-6s are considered essential to our diet, it's the ratio that matters. A high omega-6/omega-3 ratio promotes inflammation and increases the risk of other diseases.

It's possible to watch your diet, eat healthier, and focus on foods considered higher in omega-3 fatty acids. Dr. Andrew Weil has a very popular anti-inflammatory diet that, if followed, brings omega-3 and omega-6 fatty acids back into balance.

DR. WEIL'S ANTI-INFLAMMATORY DIET

Dr. Weil uses a food pyramid to demonstrate his anti-inflammatory diet. You want to eat most of the foods at the bottom (or wide part) of the pyramid and less of what is at the top (or narrow part) of the pyramid.

Dr. Weil's anti-inflammatory diet recommends three to four servings per day of **fruits** (one serving is defined as a medium piece of fruit, ½ cup of chopped fruit, or ¼ cup of dried fruit). Weil recommends four to five servings per day of **vegetables** (one serving equals 2 cups of salad greens or ½ cup cooked, raw, or juiced vegetables). Other recommendations include:

Beans and legumes: one to two servings per day (one serving equals ½ cup cooked beans or legumes)

Pasta al dente: two to three servings per week (one serving is equal to ½ cup cooked grains)

Whole and cracked grains: three to five servings a day (one serving is equal to ½ cup cooked grains)

Healthy fats: five to seven servings per day (one serving is equal to 1 teaspoon oil, two walnuts, 1 tablespoon flaxseed, 1 ounce of avocado)

Fish/Seafood: two to six servings per week (one serving is equal to 4 ounces of fish or seafood)

Whole soy foods: one to two servings per day (one serving equals ½ cup tofu or tempeh, 1 cup soymilk, ½ cup cooked edamame, 1 ounce of soynuts)

Cooked Asian mushrooms: unlimited

Other Protein Sources: one to two servings a week (one serving equals 1 ounce of cheese, an 8-ounce serving of dairy, one egg, 3 ounces cooked poultry or skinless meat)

Healthy Herbs and Spices: Unlimited

Tea: two to four cups per day

Supplements: daily, high-quality multivitamin/multimineral supplement

Red wine: optional (maximum is one or two glasses per day)

Healthy sweets: sparingly (dark chocolate is a good choice)

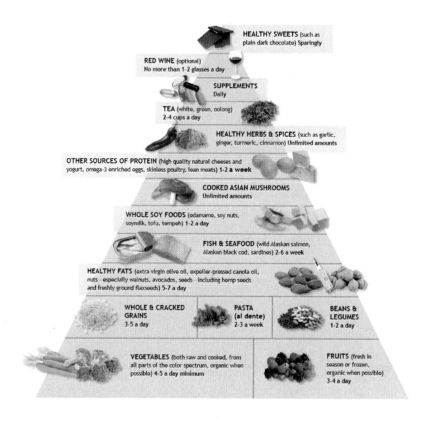

GOODBYE, USDA FOOD PYRAMID; HELLO, MYPLATE

In June 2011, the government of the United States (USDA) rolled out its new graphic to replace the well-established food pyramid for good nutrition (a different pyramid from Dr.Weil's Anti-inflammatory Food Pyramid). The USDA pyramid, known as MyPyramid, could be found at http://mypyramid.gov. The new graphic, called MyPlate, was created partly to promote Michelle Obama's war on obesity. As you know, obesity has been strongly linked to osteoarthritis.

The graphic is a plate divided into four sections, with fruits and vegetables taking up half the plate. Grains and protein make up the other half of the plate, and there is a graphic for dairy.

The message our government wants conveyed is watch your calories, eat less, and avoid oversized portions. They recommend that half of your plate be fruits and vegetables, and at least half of your grains should be whole grains. As for milk or milk products, fat-free or low-fat (1%) is your best choice. Also, be aware of the sodium content in any foods you buy. Read labels and choose low-sodium foods. Last, but not least, water is the preferred drink choice—and lots of it.[7]

CELIAC DISEASE AND GLUTEN-FREE DIET

Celiac disease has been found to occur with various auto-immune diseases. There has been a close association found between Celiac disease and Sjogren's syndrome.[8] Celiac disease is characterized by damage to the small intestine by consumption of foods that contain gluten such as wheat, barley and rye. Due to this damage, affected patients cannot absorb certain nutrients. Diagnosis my be aided by blood tests or tissue samples of the small intestine obtained during an endoscopic procedure (an endoscope is a tube with a camera that is used by a gastroenterologist to look into the stomach and small intestine and biopsy selected tissue). According to celiac.org, classic symptoms of Celiac disease include

---

7   MyPlate.gov, http://www.choosemyplate.gov/.

8   S. Iltanen et al., "Celiac Disease and Markers of Celiac Disease Latency in Patients with Primary Sjögren's Syndrome," *American Journal of Gastroenterology* 94 (1999): 1042–1046, http://www.ncbi.nlm.nih.gov/pubmed/10201480.

abdominal cramping, intestinal gas, bloating, diarrhea or constipation, fatty stools, anemia, unexplained weight loss with a large appetite, or weight gain. Joint pain, osteopenia, osteoporosis, fatigue, and depression are also linked to the condition. The only treatment for Celiac disease is a gluten-free diet, and there must be strict adherence to the diet. When gluten is removed from the diet, the small intestine starts to heal and general health improves.

Even people who have not been diagnosed with Celiac disease may benefit from a gluten-free or low-gluten diet. Dr. Zashin, based on clinical experience, suggests trying to avoid gluten for four weeks to see whether the change is helpful. This is true for any foods you suspect may be a problem. Try eliminating them from your diet for a few weeks to see whether there is noticeable improvement in your symptoms. Reintroduction of the suspected food with recurrence of symptoms can help confirm whether or not a specific food is the culprit.

THE BOTTOM LINE

Make reasonable, healthful choices when defining your diet. Make choices that would be in keeping with the anti-inflammatory diet, too, but even so, keep your expectations in check. There is no diet that promises a cure; it's just another way to help manage arthritis.

_____

Conclusion by Dr. Scott Zashin

In addition to my training at Dartmouth Medical School and residency at the University of Texas Southwestern Medical Center, one of the most important sources of learning is from my patients' experiences. As a young physician, I took care of a gentleman who was always in pain. He rarely smiled and one day came to the office smiling. When I questioned why he thought he was feeling so well, he replied, "Acupuncture!" As a result, I knew I needed to learn how to perform acupuncture. I became interested in natural treatments after using acupuncture to treat my patients with knee arthritis, back pain, and fibromyalgia.

Several years later, one of my patients with rheumatoid arthritis presented to my office with significantly less swelling and pain than on her previous visit. In fact, her inflammatory markers in the blood were also improved. It turns out she had been eating a significant number of cherries, which she felt were the reason she was so much better. I wanted to learn more about the beneficial effects of cherries to help arthritis. My research led me to Mr. Bob Underwood, a former cherry farmer from Traverse City, Michigan. Bob was aware of the benefits of Montmorency tart cherries helping people with their joint health, but unfortunately, these cherries were not always in season. After years of work, Bob developed a product called CherryFlex, which is highlighted in this book. CherryFlex is different from the cherry extracts marketed around the country in that it contains the skin and pulp of the Montmorency tart cherries.

I have used CherryFlex for more than six years in my practice to help patients with their joint issues, including those with fibromyalgia, rheumatoid arthritis, osteoarthritis, and lupus. In my experience, taking two soft gels per day helped about a third of my patients who chose this therapy. Some patients who were taking NSAIDS (nonsteroidal anti-inflammatory drugs such as ibuprofen, naproxen, Celebrex, etc.) were able to discontinue these drugs and get similar benefit with CherryFlex.

I currently follow patients who have had a positive effect and remained on the product for more than four years.

As a medical doctor, I wanted to try to validate my clinical experience with scientific data. As a result, I helped Dr. Jack Cush design a clinical study with research support from Cherry Capital Services. Dr. Cush is a world-renowned arthritis researcher who is chief of arthritis research at Baylor Medical Center in Dallas, Texas. The initial study was an open-label study in patients who had osteoarthritis of the knee. An open-label study means that both patient and doctor knew they were getting CherryFlex.

There was no placebo group. This study showed that those who took CherryFlex had significant clinical improvement in their pain. As a result of this pilot study, a very small 30-patient double-blind, placebo-controlled trial was designed and conducted by Dr. Cush with limited funding from Cherry Capital Services. This time, Dr. Cush was unable to show that the CherryFlex did any better in relieving pain than the placebo. Does this mean that CherryFlex is not effective in helping patients with joint pain? I think the answer is no. Many of my patients continue to get benefit with this supplement. A number of my patients who stopped the product when they were unsure whether they were getting benefit chose to resume treatment when their symptoms returned. Dr. Cush and I continue to recommend CherryFlex to our patients who are interested in trying a natural therapy to help the pain of their arthritis.

So while the results from this double-blind trial do not mean that Cherry Flex is ineffective, it does mean that at this time, there is no evidence the product is better than placebo in relieving the pain of osteoarthritis. Further study of CherryFlex enrolling a larger number of subjects would be useful.

For those who wish to try CherryFlex to treat their joint symptoms, I have the following recommendations:

Use the product as directed, which is two capsules per day. Because there is evidence that tart cherries may improve sleep, I encourage my patients with sleep issues to take one in the morning and one capsule two hours before bed. Otherwise, I suggest one daily for a few days, and then if tolerated, two can be taken all at once. Due to the absence of safety data, I do not recommend concentrated cherry products (eg CherryFlex; Cheribundi), SAM-e, DONA (as well as other brands of glucosamine) and Avosoy (as well as other brands of avocado soy unsaponifiables) to my patients who are children, pregnant, attempting to become pregnant or who are breast-feeding.

I always recommend consulting with your doctor first before starting any product mentioned in this book. I also recommend that if you start taking CherryFlex or any of the supplements/products mentioned in this book, that you follow up with your physician within a month if you wish to continue taking them.

Please keep in mind that just because a product is "natural" does not mean there are not potential side effects to the therapy. My suggestion is to try one product at a time and give it a reasonable time to help before switching to something else.

Thank you for your interest in this book, and I hope you will feel better very soon.

Best wishes,
Scott Zashin, MD
Clinical Professor of Medicine
University of Texas–Southwestern Medical School
Dallas, TX
Attending Physician, Texas Heath Resources
Presbyterian Hospital
Dallas, Texas

For information on how to obtain products mentioned in this book, please go to

www.NaturalArthritisTreatment.com